OXFORD MEDICAL PUBLICATIONS

Diabetes and the Heart

Diabetes and the Heart

Edited by

KENNETH G. TAYLOR

Consultant Physician, Dudley Road Hospital and
Honorary Senior Clinical Lecturer, University of Birmingham
Birmingham, UK

Oxford   New York   Tokyo
OXFORD UNIVERSITY PRESS

Oxford University Press, Great Clarendon Street, Oxford OX2 6DP
Oxford New York
Athens Auckland Bangkok Bogota Bombay Buenos Aires
Calcutta Cape Town Dar es Salaam Delhi Florence Hong Kong
Istanbul Karachi Kuala Lumpur Madras Madrid Melbourne
Mexico City Nairobi Paris Singapore Taipei Tokyo Toronto
and associated companies in
Berlin Ibadan

Oxford is a trade mark of Oxford University Press

Published in the United States
by Oxford University Press Inc., New York

© K. G. Taylor, 1987

First published in 1987 by Castle House Publications Ltd
First published in paperback in 1992 by Oxford University Press

Reprinted 1997

British Library Cataloguing in Publication Data
Diabetes and the heart.
1. Diabetes   2. Heart—Diseases
I. Taylor, K. G.
616.4'62   RC660

Library of Congress Cataloging in Publication Data
(data available)

ISBN 0 71 940114 3 (Hbk)
ISBN 0 19 263026 1 (Pbk)

Printed and bound in Great Britain by
Antony Rowe Ltd, Chippenham, Wiltshire

Dedication

To Gwen, Anne, Ruth, Marion, Lynne and Chris

Authors

Dr D.J. Betteridge, BSc, PhD, MD, MRCP, Senior Lecturer in Medicine, University College Honorary Consultant Physician, University College Hospital, London, UK.

Dr P.M. Dodson, MD, MRCP, Senior Registrar, Dudley Road Hospital, Birmingham, UK.

Dr P.J. Pacy, MD, MRCP, Honorary Senior Registrar, The Nutrition Research Group, The Clinical Research Centre, Harrow, UK.

Dr J.P.D. Reckless, MD, FRCP, Consultant Physician, Royal United Hospital, Bath, UK and Honorary Senior Lecturer in Biochemistry, University of Bath, Bath, UK.

Dr K.G. Taylor, MD, MRCP, Consultant Physician, Dudley Road Hospital, Birmingham, UK and Honorary Senior Clinical Lecturer, University of Birmingham, Birmingham, UK.

Dr S. Waldron, MRCPI, Research Fellow and Honorary Registrar, Dudley Road Hospital, Birmingham, UK.

Dr R.D.S. Watson, BSc, MD, MRCP, Consultant Cardiologist, Dudley Road Hospital, Birmingham, UK.

Acknowledgements

We are indebted to Mrs B Singh (Clinical Investigation Unit, Dudley Road Hospital) for considerable effort and patience in typing the manuscript for Chapter 4.

Contents

Introduction

Why a book tackling this subject in particular? Diabetic care has seen quite revolutionary changes in attitude in recent years as physicians have come to regard the subject as a speciality in its own right. More health districts in the UK have appointed one or more physicians specialising in diabetes and there has been bustling activity into many clinical and research aspects.

A consequence of this activity has been a much greater awareness that the problems faced by diabetic patients were not resolved by the discovery and development of pure insulin preparations or the oral agents, important as these discoveries were. At whatever age diabetes is diagnosed life expectancy is reduced due to the chronic complications, and the quality of life may be severely impaired by angina, heart failure, stroke, blindness, renal failure and neuropathy. Heart disease is a major cause of mortality and morbidity in diabetic patients and this fact alone justifies a book on the subject.

Another consequence of the increased interest has been questioning of the inevitability of chronic complications and of an attitude that frowned on considering dialysis and transplantation for patients with renal failure, or coronary artery bypass grafting for those with intractable angina, just because they were diabetic and not expected to do well. It is true that they do not do quite so well as non-diabetics, but the difference is not so great that diabetics should be excluded without very careful consideration.

The chapter on epidemiology defines the magnitude of the problem in Europe and North America, while that on the heart discusses coronary atheroma in the diabetic with an account of medical treatment of angina and the role of further investigation with stress testing and coronary angiography, and assesses data on bypass grafting. There follows a review of evidence supporting a specific diabetic heart muscle disease.

The following three chapters examine key factors in the development of the atheromatous plaque and the formation of thrombus. Research into the importance of hypertension for diabetic patients has lain dormant until recently on this side of the Atlantic. Hypertension is an established risk factor for atherosclerosis and it is more prevalent in patients with diabetes, although the precise mechanisms remain poorly understood. The question of therapy for hypertension is tackled and the concept developed that such therapy should not only be effective in treating the blood pressure but should not adversely affect blood lipids or glycaemic control.

The chapter on lipids explores another hitherto twilight area of diabetes. Altered lipid metabolism is a common feature of diabetes and may well contribute significantly to premature atherosclerosis. Awareness of this has paralleled the realisation that hyperlipidaemia is an important risk factor for atheroma in non-diabetics. It was only in the last decade that the potential dangers of having atheroma-prone diabetics on high-fat low-carbohydrate diets were fully recognised.

Platelets have emerged as a very important subject. Clearly they have an essential role in the formation of thrombus on an atheromatous plaque, but they may well be involved in the pathogenesis of the plaque itself. The diabetic state appears to affect platelet function and this chapter discusses this relatively uncharted area with potential therapeutic benefits for the future.

The book concludes with a chapter which discusses the practical management of diabetes during acute myocardial infarction and the long-term strategies to attempt to reduce the incidence of chronic complications. This raises not only questions about the best type of management but also how care should be provided and the roles of primary- and secondary-care physicians.

Although the book can be regarded as a whole, each chapter stands on its own with references for those who wish to read more extensively. All the authors are clinicians who are involved in the care of diabetic patients and research in their respective fields of special interest. Each chapter commences with a brief profile of the author so that readers may appreciate the perspective in which the chapter is written.

K.G. Taylor 1986

Chapter One

The Epidemiology of Heart Disease in Diabetes Mellitus

J.P.D. Reckless

Dr John Reckless qualified from St Bartholomew's Hospital in 1968 and returned there for a period of research work in adipose tissue and lipid metabolism. He became an MCR Travelling Fellow at the University of California, San Diego, looking at lipoprotein metabolism in cultured arterial endothelium. After senior registrar appointments at Barts and Sheffield, he is now a Consultant Physician and Endocrinologist in the Bath District and Honorary Senior Lecturer in Biochemistry at the University of Bath.

Introduction

Insulin therapy from 1922 reduced death rates in younger diabetics (Stocks, 1944), but macrovascular disease has made an increasing contribution to mortality (Marks & Krall, 1971; West, 1978 a; Krolewski, et al, 1985). Coronary artery disease is the major cause of death in the diabetic and a major cause of morbidity, forming part of the spectrum of atherosclerosis and large-vessel disease. End-organ disease is not limited to the heart however, and concomitant disease affecting the cerebral and peripheral (limb) vasculature is common, and gives rise to considerable morbidity and mortality (Warren et al, 1966; Robertson & Strong, 1968; Westlund, 1969; Bradley, 1971; National Heart, Lung and Blood Institutes, 1978; West, 1978 b, c). While one-third of North Americans will die of an atherosclerotic disease, this will be the cause of death in three-quarters of North America's diabetics (Marble, 1976; Steiner, 1981). For these reasons, and as some studies examine not just coronary artery disease but cardiovascular disease in its entirety, some consideration will be given to cerebrovascular disease and peripheral vascular disease. Macrovascular disease in the diabetic tends to follow similar patterns to disease in the non-diabetic, and accelerated, premature, or more severe atherosclerosis appears the main cause of excess disease in the diabetic (Strandness et al, 1964; Sternby, 1968). Diabetic microvascular disease, arterial medial sclerosis and calcification may coexist and complicate atherosclerotic macrovascular disease, but this review will be limited to large-vessel disease.

The predilection to macrovascular disease is not confined to a particular type of diabetes. Significant atherosclerotic lesions are not necessarily related to either duration or severity of diabetes. Macrovascular disease may be the presenting event in persons with impaired glucose tolerance (Bradley, 1971). Such early macrovascular disease in those with impaired glucose tolerance or non-insulin-dependent diabetes has also been found in prospective studies (Ostrander et al, 1974; Keen, 1976; Pirart, 1978; Fuller et al, 1979; Kannel & McGee, 1979 a), while insulin-dependent diabetics may show accelerated macrovascular disease within 10–15 years of onset of diabetes (Crall & Roberts, 1978). Besides hyperglycaemia and other metabolic and hormonal abnormalities, diabetics have an increased frequency of other potential risk factors such as hypertension, hyperlipaemia and abnormal blood coagulability, together with coexisting microvascular disease.

Consideration of macrovascular disease in the diabetic population requires comparison with either the non-diabetic population, or alternatively the general population from which the diabetic sample data derives. The high prevalence and incidence rates of coronary heart disease in general populations from developed countries have to be borne in mind in order to interpret disease frequency in diabetics. Selection of subjects included in samples is frequently prone to considerable bias, with resulting distortion of rates of macrovascular disease both in the diabetic and non-diabetic groups, and with resulting difficulty in assessing potential risk factors (Pyorala & Laasko, 1983). Definitions and diagnosis of diabetes have varied widely from study to study, from country to country, and with time. Insulin-dependent diabetes mellitus and non-insulin-dependent diabetes mellitus have not been clearly differentiated in some studies, leading to difficulties in data interpretation. Excess renovascular deaths occur particularly in insulin-dependent diabetics, but these patients may have accompanying macrovascular disease. However, as duration of diabetes increases to, and beyond, 30 years, recruitment to renovascular deaths falls for reasons that are not clearly understood. This may distort interpretation of age-related macrovascular deaths unless type and duration of diabetes are also considered.

As diabetes is associated with excess deaths from macrovascular disease, consideration of prevalence of macrovascular morbidity will tend to be an underestimate of total macrovascular disease in diabetics. Longitudinal studies (of incidence) of macrovascular disease are less likely to be influenced by this effect, while precision of identification of macrovascular disease is also likely to be better in incidence data as opposed to cross-sectional (prevalence) data. Where possible longitudinal studies, with adequate non-diabetic cohorts for comparison, will be given most prominence.

Overall Cardiovascular Mortality in Diabetes

Studies in different countries have examined mortality from cardiovascular disease in diabetics, either in diabetic populations from defined districts, or in hospital- or clinic-based groups. Those studies which base cause of death only on death certification are likely to be unreliable due to gross underreporting of diabetes mellitus (Marks & Krall, 1971; West, 1978 c; Fuller et al, 1983; Krolewski et al, 1985; Ochi et al, 1985). In one of these studies (Ochi et al, 1985), where ascertainment of diabetes in a population was felt to be high, the diabetes mortality rate (as the underlying cause of death) was 8.5 per 100 000 person-years. Diabetes was an underlying or contributory cause at a rate of 31.5 per 100 000 person-years, while the mortality rate was 82.7 per 100 000 person-years if all deaths among diabetics were counted. Diabetes was not mentioned on the certificate in 62 per cent of the 428 diabetic deaths. However, the excess mortality of insulin-dependent and non-insulin-dependent diabetics of both sexes, in Europe, North America and elsewhere, is clearly seen when compared to their respective general populations.

Europe

Diabetics from the clinic at the General Hospital, Birmingham, UK, diagnosed between 1945 and 1959, over the age of 40 years and mainly non-insulin-dependent, were studied in 1959 (Hayward & Lucena, 1965). For 2278 male diabetics there was a 1.59-fold excess of circulatory system deaths. In the 3727 female diabetics the ratio was higher at 1.81, the mortality ratio in females increasing with duration of diabetes mellitus. Presence of hypertension increased this risk in both males and females. In Oslo, 3832 newly diagnosed diabetics on discharge from hospital were identified for the years 1925–1955, and traced until 1965 (Westlund, 1969). In the whole period of study, the overall mortality ratios for all causes were increased at 2.92 for male and 2.82 for female diabetics, compared to the general population. The mortality ratio for coronary artery disease was 3.87 for males and 3.62 for females. Those who had data for the period 1951–1961 showed ratios twice those observed in Birmingham, and the relative risk ratios were higher in younger diabetics with macrovascular disease being increased and premature. Thus those male diabetics in Oslo reaching age 70 or more had a mortality ratio for coronary artery disease of 2.4 compared to the general population, while in those male diabetics failing to reach age 70 the risk ratio for mortality from coronary artery disease was higher still at 4.3. The patterns for females were similar but risks were higher, the ratio being 2.8 for those of 70 years of age or more, and 8.6 for those not attaining 70 years. This particularly increased susceptibility of younger diabetic females is found in other populations, females losing some of their relative protection compared to males.

Similar findings were obtained in a retrospective study in Warsaw, where 5261 diabetics aged 30–68 years at the time of diagnosis were followed for 1–11 years and showed an overall mortality from all causes increased 1.31-fold for males and 1.27-fold for females (Krolewski et al, 1977). Deaths from cerebrovascular disease were increased 2.95- and 1.47-fold, and from coronary artery disease 1.95- and 1.75-fold, for males and females, respectively. Relative risk ratios were higher in younger patients than older both for overall mortality and for mortality from cerebrovascular or coronary artery disease. In diabetics aged 30–49 years at diagnosis mortality ratios for coronary artery disease were 3.40 and 3.33 for males and females, respectively.

A follow-up for 1977 was carried out on 307 diabetics who had attended the Danish Steno Memorial Hospital, and who were diagnosed before 1933 at age 30 years or less (Deckert et al, 1978). Forty per cent of diabetics were alive, and the overall mortality from all causes was two to six times higher than for a control population. At a time when 10 per cent of the general population had died, 50 per cent of the diabetics were dead. Diabetics aged less than 10 years at diagnosis had a worse prognosis than those diagnosed at ages 21–30 years. Longer survival was seen in the diabetic women, which was not fully explained by the longer survival of women in general. Thirty-one per cent of deaths were due to diabetic nephropathy, while ischaemic heart disease was increased by 25 per cent.

In East Germany in a cohort of 2560 diabetics newly diagnosed in 1966, data for the 10 years 1966–1976 were studied. One thousand and fifty-four had died, 63 per cent from cardiovascular causes (Panzram & Zabel-Langhennig, 1981). Ratios expressing excess mortality (largely from increased macrovascular and ischaemic heart disease) ranged from 2.2 to 1.0 and decreased with age. The decline in relative mortality with increasing age has been demon strated in other studies (Hayward & Lucena, 1965; Gronberg et al, 1967; Westlund, 1969; Marks & Krall, 1971; Krolewski et al, 1985).

Fuller et al (1983) has examined death certification for diabetics in England and Wales for the years 1972–1977. While diabetes may often have been omitted from death certificates, deaths from ischaemic heart disease were increased 25 per cent and 40 per cent in male and female diabetics, respectively. Increases were much greater in the younger age-groups, and more so in females. Fuller et al (1983) also followed 5971 known diabetics (members of the British Diabetic Association) and traced 2134 death certificates, one-third of which did not mention diabetes. In this group mortality rates were 1.87- and 2.74-fold increased in males and females. In those aged 15–44 years rates were increased 4.98- and 11.54-fold over non-diabetics.

North America — Joslin Clinic

The most extensive follow-up studies of diabetics come from the Joslin Clinic in Boston (Marks & Krall, 1971; Krolewski et al, 1985), and show changing trends in overall- and specific-cause mortality from the time of pre-insulin therapy to about 1970. Deaths from ketoacidosis fell markedly with insulin, and have declined gradually since to about 1 per cent. The deaths in diabetics aged 40 years or more have fallen also, but less dramatically. The mortality of diabetic patients first seen at the Joslin Clinic between 1950 and 1958, and traced to 1961, have been compared to mortality in the general population (Entmacher et al, 1964; Marks, 1965), and data for different ages and sex are shown in Table 1.1. The mortality ratio was 1.6- to 7.4-fold higher in the male, and 2.4- to 13.9-fold higher in the female diabetics. The maximum ratios were reached in the group aged 25–34 years at diagnosis, and decreased gradually again with increasing age. The Joslin Clinic has also calculated life expectancy according to the age at diagnosis of

diabetes compared to that of the general population (Marks & Krall, 1971; Krolewski et al, 1985), and the data are shown in Figure 1.1. Life expectancy is reduced at all ages of onset, by the longest number of years in diabetic groups with the youngest age of onset, but by about a third at any age of onset.

Deaths from all cardiovascular and renal causes accounted for only 20 per cent of deaths in the pre-insulin period, but had risen to 75 per cent by the 1960s. Between 1956 and 1968 inclusive there were 9214 deaths and the major causes of death are shown in Table 1.2. Large-vessel disease accounts for around 70 per cent of deaths in those aged 20 years or more at onset of diabetes, and cardiac disease for more than 50 per cent. It is clear that age of onset of diabetes has a different relationship to microvascular than to macrovascular deaths. Microvascular disease is most marked in younger patients. Duration of diabetes is positively related to deaths from diabetic renal disease in patients under 40 years at diagnosis and especially in those under 20 years at diagnosis. Macrovascular disease was more common in those older than 20 years at diagnosis. The frequency of deaths from cardiac causes did increase with duration of diabetes in those with an onset of diabetes under

Table 1.1 Mortality, by age and sex, of diabetics compared with controls

Age at onset (years)	Males			Females		
	Death rate per 1000			Death rate per 1000		
	Diabetics	Controls	Ratio	Diabetics	Controls	Ratio
5–14	0.9*	0.5	1.8	0.8*	0.3	2.7
15–24	5.4*	1.2	4.5	0.8*	0.6	1.3
25–34	10.3†	1.4	7.4	15.3	1.1	13.9
35–44	16.1	3.7	4.4	10.4†	2.3	4.5
45–54	21.5	10.3	2.1	18.2	5.8	3.1
55–64	44.9	24.7	1.8	35.7	14.6	2.4
65–74	84.8	53.0	1.6	85.5	35.7	2.4

Mortality of diabetic patients first seen at the Joslin Clinic in 1950–1958 and traced to 1 January 1961, compared with mortality in the general population.
Data from Entmacher et al (1964).
*Based on less than five deaths.
†Based on five to 19 deaths.

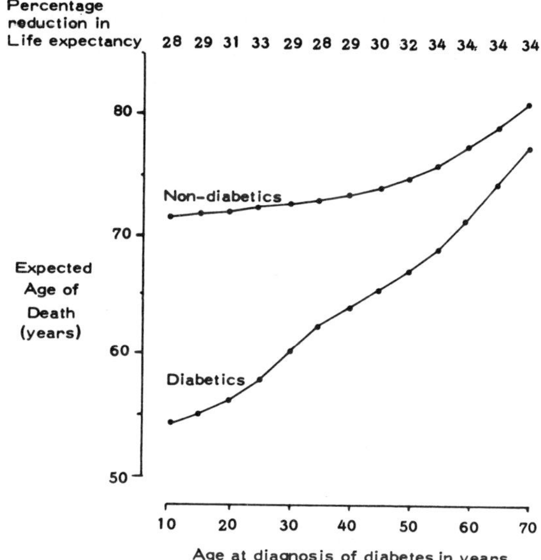

Figure 1.1 Expectation of life in diabetics and non-diabetics. For different attained ages the expected ages at death are shown for diabetics and for the general population. The relative reduction in life expectancy is shown as a percentage. Thus at any age a person developing diabetes has a life expectancy one-third less than a non-diabetic of a similar age. Values for older ages are likely to be fairly accurate, but for younger ages less so. Diabetic data exclude deaths within one week of first observation or hospital discharge. Data from the Joslin Clinic analysed by the Metropolitan Life Insurance Company. Data from Marks & Krall (1971, Tables 9–11).

40 years of age. While there is increased cardiac disease in older diabetics, there was no evidence of increasing risk with increasing duration of diabetes. The relative ratios for specific causes of cardiovascular mortality are shown in Table 1.3, there being 2.4- and 3.4-fold increases in cardiovascular disease, in males and females, respectively. In younger diabetics (15–44 years) relative risks were much higher at 12.2- and 19.5-fold for males and females respectively, this being related to the low rates of degenerative vascular, and especially cardiac, disease in the general population. Increase in cerebrovascular disease was two-fold. The excess renovascular disease reflects renal deaths in the young diabetic with long disease duration.

Atherosclerotic heart disease accounted for 50.6, 53.7 and 54.5 per cent of all diabetic deaths in the 1950s, 1960s and 1970s, respectively (Leland & Maki, 1985). While overall mortality from coronary artery disease in the USA general population reached a peak in the 1960s, it has fallen by more than 20 per cent since 1968. However, no such fall has occurred in the diabetic coronary artery disease mortality rate.

North America — other studies

In Rochester, Minnesota, of 1099 diabetics

Table 1.2 Cardiovascular causes of death, by age and sex, as a percentage of all causes of death in 9214 Joslin Clinic diabetics dying between 1956 and 1968

Cause of death	Age at onset (years)							
	Males				Females			
	<20	20–39	40–59	60+	<20	20–39	40–59	60+
Cardiovascular–renal	80	79	75	73	75	76	78	76
Macrovascular	32	62	71	70	32	62	73	73
Cardiac	26	53	57	52	25	53	56	51
Cerebral	5	7	11	13	6	7	14	18
Other*	1	2	3	5	1	2	3	4
Microvascular	48	17	4	2	43	14	6	3
Nephropathy	41	13	2	0	38	7	3	1
Other renal	6	5	2	2	6	7	3	2

*Includes diabetic gangrene and arteriosclerosis (unspecified)
Data from Marks & Krall (1971, Tables 9–16).

Table 1.3 Relative mortality from vascular causes for diabetic patients of age 15–74 years first seen in the Joslin Clinic between 1950 and 1958 and traced to 1961

Cause of death	Death rate ratios for the diabetic to general population	
	Males	Females
Total vascular disease	2.4	3.4
Aged 15–44 years	12.2	19.5
Aged 45–74 years	2.2	3.2
Heart disease	2.0	3.2
Cerebrovascular disease	1.8	2.0
Renovascular	17.8	17.0

Data from Entmacher et al (1964) and from Marks & Krall (1971, Tables 9–18).

identified from medical records for 1945–1970 there were 510 deaths, 55 per cent being from macrovascular disease (Palumbo et al, 1976). The 198 deaths in diabetics from coronary heart disease were significantly in excess of the 115 expected. In reviews of experiences in life insurance for selected diabetics increased mortality ratios of four to five were found, ratios being higher for younger insulin-treated subjects (McGurl & Pollack, 1965; Goodkin & Wolloch, 1969).

In a community-wide health survey in Washington County, 371 diabetics aged 20–75 years were identified out of a population of 26 000 (Dupree & Meyer, 1980). Over the next 39 months diabetics suffered a 2.5-fold excess mortality compared to the main population. The increase was 1.5-fold for non-insulin-dependent diabetics, but 8-fold for insulin-treated patients. This particular increase in insulin-treated patients reflects a low mortality rate for non-diabetics in this younger age-group. The excess mortality in the diabetics was due to a particular increase in vascular disease, the ratio being 4.8 overall, and 2.5 and 14.2 for non-insulin-dependent and insulin-treated diabetics respectively. Similar findings to those of Dupree and Meyer were found in a study of diabetics employed by the Du Pont Company (Pell & D'Alonzo, 1970), where

370 male diabetics were compared to a series of matched controls from the same population for their 10-year survival and for the findings at their periodic company health examinations. The diabetic death rate over 10 years was 25.4 per cent compared to 9.7 per cent in the controls, a ratio of 2.6. There was a higher prevalence of hypertension, obesity, coronary artery disease and kidney disease, while mortality was also influenced by severity of diabetes, as judged by insulin dose, age of onset, and recurrent glyco-suria. Hypertension was 1.54 times more common in the diabetics. Diabetics taking 40 or more units of insulin per day had lower absolute mortality rates than the others, reflecting their younger age, but on a matched-to-controls basis their risk was increased 5.7-fold, while risks were increased 2.5- and 2.2-fold for those on a lower insulin dose or not receiving insulin.

Other populations

In populations where coronary artery disease is uncommon, diabetics also have less coronary atheroma although still usually in excess of that in their appropriate non-diabetic population. Environmental factors affecting the whole population also seem to affect diabetics, who are more susceptible to them.

For example, coronary artery disease is an uncommon cause of death in the general population in Japan, accounting for less than 1 in 16 of diabetic deaths (Goto & Fukuhara, 1968). Japanese, in Japan, have been compared with a Japanese population in Hawaii (Kawate et al, 1979), where calorie intakes were similar but fat and refined carbohydrates were higher in Hawaii. Diabetic deaths were much higher in Japanese migrants in Hawaii. Both diabetics and non-diabetics had increased death rates from ischaemic heart disease. In Japan macrovascular disease has also been related to age and blood pressure but not to diabetic control (Ishihara et al, 1984). In a Chinese study, diabetics with a disease duration greater than 10 years had an increased mortality (Xiaoren et al, 1981).

In Puerto Rico diabetics have low rates of coronary artery disease (Gordon et al, 1974). Similar low rates are found in the populations of Central America (West & Kalbfleisch, 1970), the native New World (West, 1974) and Nigeria (Greenwood & Taylor, 1968). In Fiji (Cassidy, 1967) the Indian population of diabetics has seven times more ischaemic heart disease than do Melanesian diabetics. Studies of diabetics in various Pacific populations suggest that macrovascular disease is less common than in Caucasian diabetics (Zimmet, 1979), but does occur and may be increasing in frequency. However, in Samoa the diabetic mortality rate is even higher than in the USA (Crews & MacKeen, 1982).

In a rural Australian community, the prevalence of macrovascular disease was high (Welborn et al, 1984). Logistic regression analysis with many variables was carried out: in 179 insulin-dependent patients age was the only risk factor; in 905 non-insulin-dependent patients age, serum creatinine, diabetic control, cholesterol, high-density lipoproteins and blood pressure were related to macrovascular disease.

Overall cardiovascular mortality—conclusions

1. Diabetics have an increased mortality compared to the general population.
2. The excess diabetic mortality is largely due to increased cardiovascular disease, particularly coronary artery disease.
3. Diabetic nephropathy is a major cause of death in young insulin-dependent diabetics, particularly in the first three decades after onset of diabetes.
4. With increasing duration of diabetes in younger insulin-dependent subjects large-vessel disease and especially coronary artery disease progressively become leading causes of mortality. This group has the highest relative risk for coronary artery disease.
5. The onset of diabetes in middle or later life is associated with three-quarters of deaths being from macrovascular disease and mainly coronary artery disease. Duration of diabetes has

much less impact in this group.
6. Female diabetics lose their relative protection from coronary artery disease, with higher relative risk ratios than males. Cerebrovascular risk ratios are increased, and are similar for males and females.

Epidemiology of Coronary Artery Disease in Diabetes

Coronary atheroma at autopsy

Autopsy studies comparing diabetic coronary artery disease to controls may be difficult to interpret (see Introduction). Populations studied are often selective and comparisons open to criticism, while methods should quantify the degree of atheroma. A Swedish study (Sternby, 1968) showed increased coronary artery atherosclerosis in both male and female diabetics, and more markedly so in diabetic females younger than 70. The relative deficit of atherosclerosis seen in non-diabetic females compared to males was lost. While hypertensives had more coronary artery disease than normotensives, the excess of coronary disease in the diabetic was more evident in the normotensive rather than the hypertensive.

A World Health Organisation five-centre study (which included the Swedish data) of 17 455 deaths quantified coronary atheroma (Kagan et al, 1976; Zdanov & Vihert, 1976). Raised lesions and calcified lesions in the coronary arteries were more common in the diabetic than in the control population. Subgroups of the control group were examined — a low atherosclerosis group (dying of non-cardiovascular disease), a high atherosclerosis group (dying of cardiovascular disease), and an average atherosclerosis group (stratified to represent the overall population). Diabetics had much more extensive disease than the low and average subgroups and as much as the high subgroup of controls. Hypertensive diabetics were even more affected, while duration of diabetes and the use of insulin were also positively related to the extent of coronary artery lesions.

In the International Atherosclerosis Project, 23 000 sets of coronary arteries from 14 countries were studied by standardised techniques (Robertson & Strong, 1968). Diabetics were found to have some increase in fatty streaks, usually a marked increase in raised coronary artery lesions, an increase in haemorrhagic ulcerated or thrombotic abnormalities, and an increase in narrowed or calcified lesions. Ascertainment of diabetes mellitus was likely to have been correct but perhaps incomplete, which would have tended to underestimate excess disease in diabetics. Diabetics may have had more hypertension than non-diabetics, may have been more likely to come to postmortem, and the type of treatment and duration of diabetes were not considered. Excess disease was still seen in diabetics compared to controls if deaths from hypertensive or atherosclerotic disease were excluded from the analysis.

In another study (Waller et al, 1980), quantitative analysis of coronary artery atherosclerosis at postmortem was carried out in 64 diabetics without and 164 with clinical coronary artery disease, compared to 183 non-diabetic controls who died from coronary artery disease. Narrowing of the coronary arteries was more severe in diabetics with clinical disease than in those without. Narrowing by at least 75 per cent was similar in diabetics compared to controls, except that severe narrowing of the left main coronary artery was more common in diabetics. However, the absence of controls dying without clinical coronary artery disease limits interpretation.

A further postmortem study (Vigorita et al, 1980) of 185 diabetics and 185 matched controls examined angiographically coronary arteries fixed in distension. Diabetics had more coronary artery disease of a more diffuse nature involving more coronary vessels and with more collateral vessels. They also had more myocardial infarcts. Duration and severity of diabetes were not apparently related to extent of coronary disease. In a smaller number of patients Crall & Roberts (1978) had similar results.

Myocardial infarction at autopsy

Various studies have shown a 2-fold increase in frequency of myocardial infarction among diabetics of both sexes, even allowing for possible autopsy selection bias (Feldman & Feldman, 1954; Goldenberg et al, 1958; Sternby, 1968; Ingelfinger et al, 1976). The last study of Pima Indians differs from the others in that the population has a very high frequency of diabetes but a low risk of coronary artery disease (Ingelfinger et al, 1976). Q-wave changes in the electrocardiogram were present in 1.6 per cent of the Pima, half the rate in Tecumseh, Michigan. In those Pima Indians dying at age 40 years or more, postmortem studies show myocardial infarction to have occurred in 15 per cent of males and 8 per cent of females. Diabetics had more coronary artery disease than non-diabetics, both at postmortem and on electrocardiogram.

Clinical coronary artery disease

Prevalence

Comparisons of 35 diabetics with 77 controls undergoing coronary artery angiography for clinical coronary artery disease (Verska & Walker, 1975) suggested more severe symptoms in the diabetics for similar vessel disease. Dortimer et al (1978) found more severe coronary artery lesions in 37 diabetics compared to 79 controls. Another study (Hamby et al, 1976), comparing 100 diabetics, 100 patients with impaired glucose tolerance and 100 non-diabetic controls, showed that both glucose intolerant groups had more vessels involved and more severe stenoses. Hypertriglyceridaemia (but not hypercholesterolaemia) was more prevalent, and was partly linked to the severity of coronary artery disease. Hypertension, gout and peripheral vascular disease were also more common compared to controls.

In Finland, prevalence of angina pectoris was 1.9 times greater in diabetics than non-diabetics, matching the two-fold increase of abnormalities in ECGs analysed by the Minnesota Code

(Reunanen et al, 1979). A higher prevalence of ECG abnormalities in diabetics was also found in other studies (Ducimetiere et al, 1979; Sakuma et al, 1979; Stamler et al, 1979 a, b). Pima Indians with a very high rate of diabetes mellitus do not show as high a rate of coronary artery disease as the USA white population, but those with diabetes had rather more ECG abnormalities than those without (Ingelfinger et al, 1976). Various studies have suggested that coronary artery disease is already increased 1.4- to 4-fold at the time of diagnosis of diabetes (Keen et al, 1965; Weaver et al, 1970; Pyorala & Laasko, 1983). Interestingly, subjects in the Bedford Study (Keen et al, 1965) with previously undiagnosed impaired glucose tolerance rather than diabetes mellitus also had increased cardiovascular problems intermediate between normals and diabetics.

Prevalence data show that diabetics who are younger, diabetics with a long duration of disease, and pre-menopausal female diabetics fare relatively less well. The earlier deaths in diabetics will tend to lead to underestimates of prevalence. In a study of 832 patients consecutively hospitalised in a Danish centre (Rytter et al, 1985), the prevalence of diabetes was 9.7 per cent, higher than in the age matched population where it was 6.1 per cent ($P < 0.001$). The prevalence of diabetes was higher for women than men (14.9 : 7.6 per cent). The risk of infarction was twice as high in insulin-dependent diabetics compared to controls. It was also doubled in non-insulin-dependent diabetic women but not in non-insulin-dependent men. Furthermore, mortality of diabetics in the month after infarction was 42.0 per cent, and 20.2 per cent in non-diabetics ($P < 0.001$).

Incidence

Prospective assessments of incidence of coronary artery disease in diabetics have confirmed these risks. In the Framingham study over a 20-year period the age-adjusted total incidence rates for coronary artery disease were 24.8 for diabetic men compared to 14.9 per 1000 for non-diabetic men, and for women the rates were 17.8

compared to 6.9 per 1000 (Kannel & McGee, 1979a). A 10-year follow-up (Jarrett et al, 1982 b) of the Bedford study (Keen et al, 1965) showed two-fold increases in incidence of coronary artery disease in males with diabetes and with impaired glucose tolerance, compared to controls. Diabetic females had five times the risk of non-diabetics, while those with impaired glucose tolerance were intermediate. Whitehall civil servants (Fuller et al, 1980) with previously known diabetes and followed over 7.5 years had a two-fold increase in risk of coronary artery disease, while those newly diagnosed at entry into the study had an even greater risk. Finnish patients with previously known diabetes followed over a mean period of nine years had coronary artery disease risk ratios of 3.0 in men and 3.1 in women, and overall cardiovascular mortality risk ratios of 3.6 and 3.9, respectively (Reunanen et al, 1979; Pyorala & Laasko, 1983). In the newly diagnosed male and female diabetics, cardiovascular mortality risk ratios were 1.5 and 3.2, and coronary artery disease mortality risk ratios were 2.0 and 6.1, respectively (Reunanen et al, 1979; Pyorala & Laasko, 1983). An Israeli study of diabetic men (Herman et al, 1977) showed an observed-to-expected overall mortality ratio of 2.0, the ratios for death from myocardial infarction and for sudden death being 3.4 and 2.4, respectively. In Evans County, USA, definite diabetics had an increased cardiovascular mortality ratio of 2.5 compared to non-diabetics (Heyden et al, 1980). Ratios were similar for males and females, but numbers of deaths studied were relatively small. The particular risk in females has been confirmed in the Framingham Study over a 20-year period, male and female diabetics having 2.1- and 4.9-fold increased risks compared to controls (Garcia et al, 1974; Kannel, 1978; Kannel & McGee, 1979 a, b).

Like mortality data, the incidence data for myocardial infarction and for angina pectoris show increases in the diabetic subsets: of 1.5- and 2.6-fold in Framingham male and female diabetics (Kannel, 1978), and of 1.4- to 3-fold in all diabetics in the Israel Ischaemic Heart Disease study (Herman et al, 1977). Incidence of angina pectoris in Framingham male and female diabetics was increased 1.6 and 1.9 times. In Israel the increase was 3.2 times in previously known diabetics, but not increased in newly diagnosed subjects followed for five years.

Epidemiology of Coronary Artery Disease Risk Factors in Diabetes

Many risk factors for coronary artery disease have been identified in the general population, of which lipid and lipoprotein concentrations, hypertension, smoking and diabetes mellitus are major factors. Physical activity and obesity (perhaps centripetal as opposed to centrifugal) also may be important. Macrovascular disease in diabetics could be increased because (*a*) diabetes may increase the other known risk factors directly, (*b*) the importance of the risk factors may be greater in diabetics, (*c*) diabetes may inherently increase risk independent or partly independent of the usual risk factors, (*d*) unrecognised risk factors may be linked with diabetes, or (*e*) treatment of diabetes may exacerbate the risk.

Lipids and lipoproteins

In most studies diabetics have been found to have more hypertriglyceridaemia and hyper-cholesterolaemia than controls (Saudek & Young, 1981), and this is in part due to an increase in triglyceride-rich lipoproteins. Improvement in diabetic control and reduced hyperglycaemia is usually 'accompanied by a reduction in plasma lipid levels (Tamborlane et al, 1979; Sosenko et al, 1980; Reckless et al, 1982), by reduced concentrations of very low density (VLDL) and low density (LDL) lipoproteins, by increased high density lipoproteins (HDL) and by an increase in the HDL subfraction HDL_2 (Reckless et al, 1982; J.P.D. Reckless et al, unpublished data). Kannel & McGee (1979 b) have calculated standardised coefficients for the regression on initial choles-

terol of subsequent cardiovascular disease in the Framingham population, and suggested that the influence of plasma cholesterol as a risk factor is similar in non-diabetics and diabetics. The protective effect of higher HDL levels has been shown in females (Gordon et al, 1977), but not reported for male diabetics in this population.

In a prevalence study (Reckless et al, 1978), cardiovascular disease in insulin-dependent diabetics was associated with higher plasma cholesterol and LDL-cholesterol levels, but not with lower HDL-cholesterol levels, and this relationship was confirmed by standardised regression coefficients. In non-insulin-dependent diabetics cardiovascular disease was inversely associated with HDL and not with LDL levels, but in the insulin-dependent diabetic LDL was the significant association. The inverse relationship between HDL and cardiovascular disease was found for female patients, but for males the positive association with LDL was dominant.

Lower HDL, and HDL_2, levels have usually been found in both male and female non-insulin-dependent diabetics (Eder, 1980; Taskinen et al, 1982). As in the general population (Miller & Miller, 1975), lower HDL concentrations have been inversely associated with hypertriglyceri-daemia (Salter et al, 1981), while the triglyceride content of the HDL itself may be increased (Schonfeld et al, 1974; Aro et al, 1981). There may be links between increased plasma trigly-cerides, reduced HDL concentrations, and impaired heparin-releasable lipoprotein lipase activity (Taskinen et al, 1982). Elevated plasma triglyceride concentrations have frequently been found (Gordon et al, 1977; Mattock et al, 1979; Heyden et al, 1980; Taskinen et al, 1982), but not invariably (Taylor et al, 1981) in non-insulin-dependent diabetics, especially females.

Hypertension

Most studies have shown an association of hypertension with diabetes (Ostrander et al, 1965; Pell & D'Alonzo, 1967; Garcia et al, 1974; Ingelfinger et al, 1976; Heyden et al, 1980; Jarrett et al, 1982 a). Pell & D'Alonzo (1967) showed a 1.54-fold increase in prevalence of hypertension in diabetics. They and others (Medalie et al, 1975) have shown also a higher prevalence of hypertension among subjects who subsequently develop diabetes. In the Whitehall study (Jarrett et al, 1982 a) mean systolic and diastolic blood pressures were little different between normals and established diabetics, but newly diagnosed diabetics and those with impaired glucose tolerance were more hypertensive. Examination of blood pressures in relation to age and duration of diabetes (Goodkin, 1975; Aromaa, 1981; Christlieb et al, 1981; Pyorala & Laasko, 1983) suggests there may be a particularly increased relative risk in younger diabetics (Table 1.4), and associated with longer duration of diabetes. This suggests that the hypertension in this group is renal in origin, related to diabetic glomerulosclerosis (Aromaa, 1981; Pyorala & Laasko, 1983). Whether the hypertension has an increased cardiovascular risk in diabetics compared to non-diabetics is not clear (Pell & D'Alonzo, 1967; Goodkin, 1975; Kannel & McGee, 1979 b; Aromaa, 1981; Christlieb et al, 1981; Pyorala & Laasko, 1983), but effective treatment of hypertension may slow the decline in renal function in patients with established diabetic renal disease (Pell & D'Alonzo, 1967).

Smoking

Epidemiological relationships between smoking and specific diabetic populations have not been adequately studied, but cigarette smoking habits in diabetics appear not to have clear differences from non-diabetics (Mogensen, 1982), and the risks of smoking in diabetics appear to be similar to the risks in non-diabetics (Kannel & McGee, 1979 b). Smoking is associated with increased risk in men for cerebrovascular disease, and in both sexes for peripheral vascular disease (Gordon & Kannel, 1972).

Table 1.4 Risk ratios for the association of hypertension with diabetes at different ages

| | Risk ratios (diabetics/non-diabetics) | | | | | |
| | Males | | | Females | | |
Age (years)	DBP >100	SBP >170 DBP >100	SBP >170 DBP >100 Drug Rx	DBP >100	SBP >170 DBP >100	SBP >170 DBP >100 Drug Rx
20–29	9.13	21.58	21.58	—	—	—
30–39	3.06	2.78	2.61	2.55	6.35	5.90
40–49	2.78	4.01	4.11	1.15	1.48	2.68
50–59	2.02	2.28	2.27	1.45	1.34	2.06
60–69	1.43	1.87	2.12	1.52	1.58	1.71
70–79	1.29	1.54	1.64	0.88	0.88	1.26

Data from the Finnish Social Insurance Institution's Study population comprising 363 diabetic men, 23 453 non-diabetic men, 408 diabetic women and 19 624 non-diabetic women (Aromaa, 1981; Pyorala & Laasko, 1983).

Ratios are calculated for different age-groups for the prevalence of hypertension in diabetics compared to non-diabetics.

DBP > 100   Diastolic pressure equal to or greater than 100 mmHg.

SBP > 170   Systolic pressure equal to or greater than 170 mmHg, and diastolic pressure equal to or greater
DBP > 100   than 100 mmHg.

SBP > 170   Systolic pressure equal to or greater than 170 mmHg, and diastolic pressure equal to or
DBP > 100   greater than 100 mmHg; or patient on drug treatment for hypertension.
Drug Rx

Obesity

Obesity might be expected to have an impact on cardiovascular disease and particularly on coronary artery disease in diabetes because of the associations of obesity with non-insulin-dependent diabetes, lipid abnormalities and hypertension. Diabetics who were 20 per cent overweight in Birmingham (Hayward & Lucena, 1965) did not show excess overall mortality, while in the Du Pont Company (Pell & D'Alonzo, 1970) being 30 per cent overweight did increase coronary artery disease mortality. Calculation of standardised regression coefficients for the Framingham population did not show an increased effect of body weight on cardiovascular disease incidence for diabetics compared to non-diabetics (Kannel & McGee, 1979 b). Recently, the distribution of adiposity has received attention; obesity of the trunk and particularly intra-abdominal fat may be associated with insulin resistance and diabetes mellitus, and be a strong coronary artery disease risk.

Diabetes mellitus

In a diabetic population the presence of diabetes itself may be an independent risk factor for the development of macrovascular disease after allowance has been made for the other known risk factors. Diabetes may have no direct interaction with the major risk factors for coronary artery disease (high plasma cholesterol, blood pressure, smoking and obesity), although the position in respect of HDL and triglycerides is less clear. In Framingham studies (Garcia et al 1974; Kannel, 1978; Kannel & McGee, 1979 a, b), and in Israel (Goldbourt et al, 1975; Medalie, 1979), multivariate analyses of general populations has identified diabetes as an independent risk. In Framingham the diabetic risk was greater for females, although this particular excess was partly related to a dependent effect linked to other risk factors (Kannel, 1978). The independent risk of diabetes persisted when HDL was also included in the multivariate analysis (Gordon et al, 1977). The Framingham

study, and the Evans County study (Heyden et al, 1980), tended to examine older diabetics with a preponderance of non-insulin-dependent patients; adequate data as to whether diabetes *per se* is an independent risk factor for younger insulin-dependent diabetics are not available. However, it has also been suggested that cultural or ethnic factors are more important determinants of atherosclerosis in diabetic subjects than is the diabetic state *per se* (Keen & Jarrett, 1979; Jarrett, 1984).

Hyperinsulinaemia and hyperglycaemia

Measures of diabetic control and type of therapy have not clearly been related to excess vascular disease risk, but high blood glucose and insulin levels might have atherogenic actions on the vessel wall (Ganda, 1980). Prevalence studies (Kashyap et al, 1970; Santen et al, 1972) have found higher insulin concentrations in diabetics with macrovascular disease. However, in Bedford a low plasma insulin level two hours after a glucose load was associated with an increased risk of vascular disease over a 10-year follow-up (Jarrett et al, 1982 b).

The relationships between insulin levels and coronary heart disease in general populations have been in males (Hockaday, 1985; Welborn, 1985), but a similar relationship has not been reported in females (Welborn, 1985).

Sulphonylureas

In the USA the University Group Diabetes Program (UGDP) trial compared four different therapies (of tolbutamide, phenformin, fixed-dose insulin and variable-dose insulin) against placebo for efficacy in preventing cardiovascular complications (University Group Diabetes Program, 1970, 1975). Tolbutamide and phenformin appeared to be associated with increased cardiovascular disease, although re-analyses of the data have cast some doubt on these findings which have not been supported by other studies (Fuller, 1983), which have shown contrary findings. In Framingham female diabetics treated with insulin had the greatest cardiovascular mortality (Garcia et al, 1974), and acute myocardial infarction was twice as frequent in insulin-treated diabetics than in non-diabetics. This was not seen in non-insulin-dependent diabetics. The World Health Organisation autopsy study (Zdanov & Vihert, 1976) suggested more coronary atheroma in insulin-treated diabetics than in those on a diet or on oral hypoglycaemic agents. In Finland (Pyorala & Laasko, 1983) the age-adjusted coronary artery disease mortality risk ratios for insulin-treated diabetics to non-diabetics were 4.6 in men and 12.9 in women. In comparison, the risks for male and female diabetics treated with oral hypoglycaemic drugs or diet alone were increased only two to three times compared to non-diabetics.

The finding of a flush in some diabetics given chlorpropamide was originally suggested to have a dominant single-gene inheritance, to be preventable in some by the prostaglandin synthetase inhibitor indomethacin, and to be associated with reduced macrovascular disease (Leslie et al, 1979; Pyke, 1979; Barnett & Pyke, 1980; Barnett et al, 1980). These associations have been questioned and other studies have failed to confirm the findings (Mann & Houston, 1983).

Macrovascular Disease Associated with Coronary Artery Disease in Diabetes

Often associated with excess coronary artery disease, diabetics have increased abdominal aortic atheroma and increased aortic calcification. These risks are increased by coexisting hypertension (Zdanov & Vihert, 1976). Raised aortic lesions (Robertson & Strong, 1968), iliofemoral atheroma (Sternby, 1968) and medial calcification in younger diabetics (Root, 1949) are all more common. Claudication is increased 4-fold in diabetic men and 6-fold in diabetic women (Kannel & McGee, 1979 a), a greater excess than for other Framingham endpoints. Arterial occlusion below the knee is increased (Strandness et al, 1964; Barner et al, 1971), and gangrene is around 60 times more likely than in non-diabetics (Bell, 1952).

As with coronary artery disease there is increased risk of cerebrovascular atheroma of about 2-fold, which is less marked in the older diabetic (Baker et al, 1961; Grunnet, 1963; Sternby, 1968; Goto et al, 1974). Interestingly, the excess risk is more marked in those with normal rather than raised blood pressure (Sternby, 1968). Age-adjusted rates in Framingham were 2.5 times higher in men and 3.6 times higher in females, similar to risks for coronary artery disease (Fuller et al, 1983). When adjusted for other risk factors, the diabetes risk ratio at 2.1 remained elevated. As well as coronary artery disease, cerebrovascular disease was increased in diabetics in England and Wales compared to the general population in the death certification study of Fuller et al (1983), and in the British Diabetic Association cohort also studied.

Epidemiology of Macrovascular Disease in Non-Diabetics with Relative Hyperglycaemia and Hyperinsulinaemia

Examination of general populations, excluding known diabetics, has indicated an excess of large-vessel disease accompanying impaired glucose tolerance, or occurring in those subjects whose glucose values (random or postglucose-loading) were in the top quintile or centile of the distribution (Keen et al, 1965; Ostrander et al, 1965). Data from prospective studies over 10 or 7 years confirmed this (Epstein, 1972; Jarrett et al, 1982 b). In the Framingham study, where random or 'casual' glucose levels were measured, coronary artery disease incidence increased considerably in relation to glucose levels greater than 6.6 mmol/l (Framingham Study, 1970), independent of blood pressure, cholesterol concentration and cigarette smoking (Gordon & Kannel, 1972). In subsequent studies using various protocols results have been somewhat less clear (Stamler & Stamler, 1979). The prevalence data fairly consistently show excess electrocardiographic abnormalities in those with glucose values in the top 20 per cent of the distribution and particularly in the top 2–5 per cent, but after multivariate analysis for other risk factors such as hypertension and adiposity the independent relationship was largely lost. In the prospective studies clear excess mortality from coronary artery disease in subjects in the top quintile, or top centile, was only seen in a third, or a half, respectively, of the studies. After multivariate analyses the hyperglycaemic risk was usually lost.

Insulin itself may affect atherogenesis (Stout, 1981), potentially influencing smooth muscle cell proliferation, stimulating lipogenesis, inhibiting lipolysis, and perhaps increasing very low density lipoprotein synthesis and secretion. Prospective studies (Pyorala, 1979; Welbourn & Wearne, 1979; Ducimetiere et al, 1980; Pyorala et al, 1982) have showed positive associations between hyperinsulinaemia and coronary artery disease independent of other risk factors, particularly in respect of poststimulatory insulin levels one and two hours after a glucose load rather than in respect of fasting insulin concentrations. How relative hyperinsulinaemia is linked to coronary artery disease is unclear, but insulin resistance may be an early feature of altered carbohydrate metabolism.

Summary

This review has considered macrovascular coronary artery disease in diabetes mellitus largely from an epidemiological viewpoint. Mortality in diabetes mellitus in most western populations is usually due to macrovascular disease, and indeed over half of diabetic deaths are due to coronary artery disease. The relationships between diabetes, as a specific risk factor, and other risk factors operating in the general population has been considered. The particular susceptibility of the diabetic female compared to her non-diabetic counterpart is clear. Some of this excess risk is also apparent in persons with impaired glucose tolerance rather than overt diabetes mellitus. The features of diabetic coronary artery disease, potential reasons for these problems, and possibilities for their further investigation and potential treatment and prevention, are the subjects of later chapters in this book.

References

Aro, A., Voutilainen, E., Uusitupa, M. et al (1981). Abnormalities of serum and lipoprotein lipids in newly diagnosed type 2 diabetes. *Diabetologia* 21, 244.

Aromaa, A. (1981) *Epidemiology and Public Health Impact of High Blood Pressure in Finland.* Helsinki, Kansanelakelaitoksen Julkaisuja, A L, p. 17. (See Pyorala and Laasko (1983).)

Baker, A.B., Kinnard, J. and Iannone, A. (1961). Cerebrovascular disease: role of nutritional factors. *Neurology* 11, 380–389.

Barner, H.B., Kaiser, G.C. and Willman, V.L. (1971). Blood flow in the diabetic leg. *Circulation* 43, 391–394.

Barnett, A.H. and Pyke, D.A. (1980). Chlorpropamide-alcohol flushing and large vessel disease in non-insulin dependent diabetes. *Br. Med. J.* 2, 261–262.

Barnett, A.H., Spiliopoulos, A.J. and Pyke, D.A. (1980). Blockade of chlorpropamide-alchohol flushing by indomethacin suggests an association between prostaglandins and diabetic vascular complications. *Lancet* ii, 164–166.

Bell, E.T. (1952). A postmortem study of vascular disease in diabetics. *Arch. Pathol.* 53, 444–455.

Bradley, R.F. (1971). Cardiovascular disease. In Marble, A., White, P., Bradley, R.F. and Krall, L.P. (eds), *Joslin's Diabetes Mellitus,* Philadelphia, Lea & Febiger 11th edn, pp. 417–477.

Cassidy, J.T. (1967). Diabetes in Fiji. *N.Z. Med. J.* 66, 167–172.

Christlieb, A.R., Warram, J.A., Krolewski, A.S. et al (1981). Hypertension: the major risk factor in juvenile-onset insulin dependent diabetics. *Diabetes* 30, Suppl. 2, 90–96.

Crall, F.V. and Roberts, W.C. (1978). The extramural and intramural coronary arteries in juvenile diabetes mellitus. Analysis of nine necropsy patients aged 19–38 years with onset of diabetes before age 15 years. *Am. J. Med.* 64, 221–230.

Crews, D.E. and MacKeen, P.C. (1982). Mortality related to cardiovascular disease and diabetes mellitus in a modernizing population. *Soc. Sci. Med.* 16, 175–181.

Deckert, T., Poulsen, J.E. and Larsen, M. (1978). Prognosis of diabetics with diabetes onset before the age of thirty-one. I: Survival, causes of death, and complications. *Diabetologia* 14, 363–370.

Dortimer, A.C., Shenoy, P.N., Shiroff, R.A. et al (1978). Diffuse coronary artery disease in diabetic patients. Fact or fiction? *Circulation* **57**, 133–136.

Ducimetiere, P., Eschwege, E., Papoz, L. et al (1980). Relationship of plasma insulin levels to the incidence of myocardial infarction and coronary heart disease mortality in a middle aged population. *Diabetologia* **19**, 205–210.

Ducimetiere, P., Eschwege, E., Richard, J. et al (1979). Relationship of glucose tolerance to prevalence of ECG abnormalities and to annual mortality from cardiovascular disease: results of the Paris prospective study. *J. Chronic Dis.* **32**, 759–766.

Dupree, E.A. and Meyer, M.B. (1980). Role of risk factors in complications of diabetes mellitus. *Am. J. Epidemiol.* **112**, 100–112.

Eder, H.A. (1980). Lipid metabolism in diabetes. In *The Role of Sulphonylureas in the Treatment of Insulin Dependent Diabetes,* New York, Science & Medicine, p. 13.

Entmacher, P.S., Root, H.F. and Marks, H.H. (1964). Longevity of diabetic patients in recent years. *Diabetes* **13**, 373–377.

Epstein, F.H. (1972). Glucose intolerance and coronary heart disease incidence; recent observations. *Horm. Metab. Res.* Suppl. 4, 174–180.

Feldman, M. and Feldman, M. (1954). The association of coronary occlusion and infarction with diabetes mellitus. A necropsy study. *Am. J. Med. Sci.* **228**, 53–56.

Framingham Study (1970) *Framingham Study—16 Year Follow-up.* An epidemiological investigation of cardiovascular disease: some characteristics related to the incidence of cardiovascular disease and death. Washington DC, US Government Printing Office, Section 26.

Fuller, J.H. (1983) Clinical trials in diabetes mellitus. In Mann, J.I., Pyorala, K. and Teuscher, A. (eds), *Diabetes in Epidemiological Perspective,* London, Churchill Livingstone, pp. 265–285.

Fuller, J.H., Elford, J., Goldblatt, P. et al (1983). Diabetes mortality: new light on an underestimated public health problem. *Diabetologia* **24**, 336–341.

Fuller, J.H., McCartney, P., Jarrett, R. et al (1979) Hyperglycaemia and coronary heart disease: the Whitehall study. *J. Chronic Dis.* **32**, 721–728.

Fuller, J.H., Shipley, M.J., Rose, G. et al. (1980) Coronary heart disease risk and impaired glucose tolerance. *Lancet* **i**, 1373–1376.

Ganda, O.P. (1980) Pathogenesis of macrovascular disease in the human diabetic. *Diabetes* **29**, 931–942.

Garcia, M.J., McNamara, P.M., Gordon, T. et al (1974). Morbidity and mortality in diabetics in the Framingham population. Sixteen year follow up study. *Diabetes* **23**, 105–111.

Goldbourt, U., Medalie, J.H. and Neufeld, H.N. (1975). Clinical myocardial infarction over a five year period; III. A multivariate analysis of incidence, the Israel ischemic heart disease study. *J. Chronic Dis.* **28**, 217–237.

Goldenberg, S., Alex, M. and Blumenthal, H.T. (1958). Sequelae of arteriosclerosis of the aorta and coronary arteries. A statistical study in diabetes mellitus. *Diabetes* **7**, 98–108.

Goodkin, G. (1975). Mortality factors in diabetes. *J. Occup. Med.* **17**, 716–721.

Goodkin, G. and Wolloch, L.B. (1969). Longevity of diabetics. *J. Occup. Med.* **11**, 522–532.

Gordon T., Castelli, W.P., Hjortland, M.C. et al (1977). Diabetes, blood lipids, and the role of obesity in coronary heart disease for women. The Framingham study. *Ann. Intern. Med.* **87**, 393–397.

Gordon, T., Garcia-Palmieri, M.R., Kagan, A. et al (1974). Differences in coronary heart disease in Framingham, Honolulu and Puerto Rico. *J. Chronic Dis.* **27**, 329–344.

Gordon, T. and Kannel, W.B. (1972). Predisposition to atherosclerosis in the head, heart and legs. *J. Am. Med. Assoc.* **221**, 661–666.

Goto, Y. and Fukuhara, N. (1968). Causes of death in 933 diabetic autopsy cases. *J. Jap. Diabetic Soc.* **11**, 197.

Goto, Y., Sato, S. and Masuda, M. (1974). Cause of death in 3151 diabetic autopsy cases. *Tohoku J. Exp. Med.* **112**, 339–353.

Greenwood, B.M. and Taylor, J.R. (1968). The complications of diabetes in Nigerians. *Trop. Geogr. Med.* **20**, 1–12.

Gronberg, A., Larsson, T. and Jung, J. (1967). Diabetes in Sweden: a clinico-statistical, epidemiological and genetic study of hospital patients and death certificates. *Acta Med. Scand.* Suppl. **477**, 1–275.

Grunnet, M.L. (1963). Cerebrovascular disease: diabetes and cerebral atherosclerosis. *Neurology* **13**, 486–491.

Hamby, R.I., Sherman, L., Mehta, J. et al (1976). Reappraisal of the role of the diabetic state in coronary artery disease. *Chest* **70**, 251–257.

Hayward, R.E. and Lucena, B.C. (1965). An investigation into the mortality of diabetics. *J. Inst. Actuaries* **91**, 286–315.

Herman, J.B., Medalie, J.H. and Goldbourt, U. (1977). Differences in cardiovascular morbidity and mortality between previously known and newly diagnosed adult diabetics. *Diabetologia* **13**, 229–234.

Heyden, S., Heiss, G., Bartel, A.G. et al (1980). Sex differences in coronary mortality among diabetics in Evans County, Georgia. *J. Chronic Dis.* **33**, 265–273.

Hockaday, T.D.R. (1985). Macrovascular disease in Caucasoid diabetic patients. *Diabetologia* **28**, 385.

Ingelfinger, J.A., Bennett, P.H., Liebow, I.M. et al (1976). Coronary heart disease in the Pima Indians. Electrocardiographic findings and postmortem evidence of myocardial infarction in a population with a high prevalence of diabetes mellitus. *Diabetes* **25**, 561–565.

Ishihara, M., Yukimura, Y., Yamada, T. et al (1984). Diabetic complications and their relationships to risk factors in a Japanese population. *Diabetes Care* **7**, 533–538.

Jarrett, R.J. (1984). Type 2 (non-insulin dependent) diabetes mellitus and coronary heart disease — chicken, egg or neither? *Diabetologia* **26**, 99–102.

Jarrett, R.J., Keen, H. and Chakrabarti, R. (1982 a). Diabetes, hyperglycaemia and arterial disease. In Keen, H. and Jarrett, R.J. (eds), *Complications of Diabetes*, London, Arnold, pp. 179–203.

Jarrett, R.J., McCartney, P. and Keen, H. (1982 b). The Bedford survey: ten year mortality rates in newly diagnosed diabetics, borderline diabetics and normoglycaemic controls and risk indices for coronary heart disease in borderline diabetics. *Diabetologia* **22**, 79–84.

Kagan, A.R., Uemera, K., Sternby, N.H. et al (1976). Atherosclerosis: A five centre study. *Bull. W.H.O.* **53**, 485–546.

Kannel, W.B. (1978). Role of diabetes in cardiac diseases: conclusions from population studies. In Zoneraich, S. (ed.) *Diabetes and the Heart*, Thomas, Illinois, Springfield, pp. 97–112.

Kannel, W.B. and McGee, D.L. (1979 a). Diabetes and cardiovascular disease. The Framingham study. *J. Am. Med. Assoc.* **241**, 2035–2038.

Kannel, W.B. and McGee, D.L. (1979 b). Diabetes and cardiovascular risk factors: the Framingham study. *Circulation*, **59**, 8–13.

Kashyap, M.L., Magill, F., Rojas, L. et al (1970). Insulin and non-esterified fatty acid metabolism in asymptomatic diabetics and atherosclerotic subjects. *Can. Med. Assoc. J.* **102**, 1165–1169.

Kawate, R., Yamakido, M., Nishimoto, Y. et al (1979). Diabetes mellitus and its vascular complications in Japanese migrants on the island of Hawaii. *Diabetes Care* **2**, 161–170.

Keen, H. (1976). Glucose intolerance, diabetes mellitus and atherosclerosis; prospects for prevention. *Postgrad. Med. J.* **52**, 445–451.

Keen, H. and Jarrett, R.J. (1979). The WHO multi-national study of vascular disease in diabetes: 2. Macrovascular disease prevalence. *Diabetes Care* **2**, 187–201.

Keen, H., Rose, G., Pyke, D.A. et al (1965). Blood sugar and arterial disease. *Lancet* **ii**, 505–508.

Krolewski, A.S., Czyzyk, A., Janeczko, D. et al (1977). Mortality from cardiovascular diseases among diabetics. *Diabetologia* **13**, 345–350.

Krolewski, A.S., Warram, J.H. and Christlieb, A.R. (1985). Onset, course, complications, and prognosis of diabetes mellitus. In Marble, A., Krall, L.P., Bradley, R.F., Christlieb, A.R. and Soeldner, J.S. (eds) *Joslin's Diabetes Mellitus*, Philadelphia, Lea & Febiger, 12th edn pp. 251–277.

Leland, O.S. and Maki, P.C. (1985). Heart disease and diabetes. In Marble, A., Krall, L.P., Bradley, R.F. et al (eds), *Joslin's Diabetes Mellitus*, Philadelphia, Lea & Febiger, 12th edn, pp. 555–556.

Leslie, R.D.G., Barnett, A.H. and Pyke, D.A. (1979). Chlorpropamide-alcohol flushing and diabetic retinopathy. *Lancet* **i**, 997–999.

Mann, J.I. and Houston, A.C. (1983). The aetiology of non-insulin-dependent diabetes mellitus. In Mann, J.I., Pyorala K. and Teuscher, A. (eds), *Diabetes in Epidemiological Perspective*, London, Churchill Livingstone, pp. 122–156.

Marble, A. (1976). Late complications of diabetes: a continuing challenge. *Diabetologia* **12**, 193–199.

Marks, H.H. (1965). Longevity and mortality of diabetics. *Am. J. Public Health* **55**, 416–423.

Marks, H.H. and Krall, L.P. (1971). Onset, course, prognosis and mortality in diabetes mellitus. In Marble, A., White, P., Bradley, R.F. and Krall, L.P. (eds). *Joslin's Diabetes Mellitus*, Philadelphia, Lea & Febiger, 11th edn, pp. 209–254.

Mattock, M.B., Fuller, J.H., Maude, P.S. et al (1979). Lipoproteins and plasma cholesterol esterification in normal and diabetic subjects. *Atherosclerosis* **34**, 437–449.

McGurl, T.J. and Pollack, A.A. (1965). Diabetes mellitus experience 1951–1962. *Trans. Assoc. Life Ins. Med. Dir. Am.* **74**, 126–133.

Medalie, J.H. (1979). Risk factors other than hyperglycemia in diabetic macrovascular disease. *Diabetes Care* **2**, 77–84.

Medalie, J.H., Papier, C.M., Goldbourt, U. et al (1975). Major factors in the development of diabetes mellitus in 10000 men. *Arch. Intern. Med.* **135**, 811–817.

Miller, G.J. and Miller, N.E. (1975). Plasma high density lipoprotein concentration and development of ischaemic heart disease. *Lancet* **i**, 16–19.

Mogensen, C.E. (1982). Longterm antihypertensive treatment inhibiting progression of diabetic nephropathy. *Br. Med. J.* **285**, 685–688.

The National Heart, Lung and Blood Institutes (1978). *Fact Book for Fiscal Year 1977*. Washington DC, US DHEW publication (NIH 78 1419).

Ochi, J.W., Melton, L.J., Palumbo, P.J. et al (1985). A population-based study of diabetes mortality. *Diabetes Care* **8**, 224–229.

Ostrander, L.D., Francis, T., Hayner, N.S. et al (1965).

The relationship of cardiovascular disease to hyperglycaemia. *Ann. Intern. Med.* **62**, 1188–1198.

Ostrander, L.D., Lamphier, D.E., Block, W.D. et al (1974). Biochemical precursors of atherosclerosis: studies in apparently healthy men in a general population. *Arch. Intern. Med.* **134**, 224–230.

Palumbo, P.J., Elveback, L.R., Chu, C-P., et al (1976). Diabetes mellitus: incidence, prevalence, survivorship, and causes of death in Rochester, Minnesota, 1945–1970. *Diabetes* **25**, 566–573.

Panzram, G. and Zabel-Langhennig, R. (1981). Prognosis of diabetes mellitus in a geographically defined population. *Diabetologia* **20**, 587–591.

Pell, S. and D'Alonzo, C.A. (1967). Some aspects of hypertension in diabetes mellitus. *J. Am. Med. Assoc.* **202**, 104–110.

Pell, S. and D'Alonzo, C.A. (1970). Factors associated with long-term survival of diabetics. *J. Am. Med. Assoc.* **214**, 1833–1840.

Pirart, J. (1978). Diabetes mellitus and its degenerative complications: a prospective study of 4,400 patients observed between 1947 and 1973. *Diabetes Care* **1**, 168–188, 252–263.

Pyke, D.A. (1979). Diabetes: the genetic connections. *Diabetologia* **17**, 333–343.

Pyorala, K. (1979). Relationship of glucose tolerance and plasma insulin to the incidence of coronary heart disease: results from two population studies in Finland. *Diabetes Care* **2**, 131–141.

Pyorala, K. and Laasko, M. (1983). Macrovascular disease in diabetes mellitus. In Mann, J.I., Pyorala, K. and Teuscher, A. (eds), London, Churchill Livingstone, pp. 183–247.

Pyorala, K., Savolainen, E., Kaukola, S. et al (1982). High plasma insulin as coronary heart disease risk factor. In Eschwege, E. (ed.) *Advances in Diabetes Epidemiology*, INSERM symposium 22, Amsterdam, Elsevier Biomedical Press, p. 143.

Reckless, J.P.D., Betteridge, D.J., Wu P. et al (1978). High density and low density lipoproteins and prevalence of vascular disease in diabetes mellitus. *Br. Med. J.* **1**, 883–886.

Reckless, J.P.D., Campbell, R.R., Betteridge, D.J. et al (1982). Effects of improved diabetic control on lipoprotein concentrations and platelet-specific proteins. *Diabetologia* **23**, 195.

Reckless, J.P.D., Campbell, R.R., Betteridge, D.J. Favourable effects on lipoprotein concentrations of improved diabetic control in short and long term. Unpublished observations.

Reunanen, A., Pyorala, K., Aromaa, A. et al (1979). Glucose tolerance and coronary heart disease in middle-aged Finnish men: Social Insurance Institution's coronary heart disease study. *J. Chronic Dis.* **32**, 747–758.

Robertson, W.B. and Strong, J.P. (1968). Athero-sclerosis in persons with hypertension and diabetes mellitus. *Lab. Invest.* **18**, 538–551.

Root, H.F. (1949). Diabetes and vascular disease in youth. *Am. J. Med. Sci.* **217**, 545–553.

Rytter, L., Troelsen, S. and Beck-Nielsen, H. (1985). Prevalence and mortality of acute myocardial infarction in patients with diabetes. *Diabetes Care* **8**, 230–234.

Sakuma, K., Hashimoto, T., Maeda, Y. et al (1979). Report on hyperglycemia in middle-aged male Japanese national railway workers. *J. Chronic Dis.* **32**, 779–786.

Salter, A.M., Mattock, M., Fuller, J.H. et al (1981). High density lipoprotein subfractions in non-insulin-dependent diabetes. *Diabetologia* **21**, 322–323.

Santen, R.J., Willis, P.W. and Fajans, S.S. (1972). Atherosclerosis in diabetes mellitus. *Arch. Intern. Med.* **130**, 833–843.

Saudek, C.D. and Young, N.L. (1981). Cholesterol metabolism in diabetes mellitus: the role of diet. *Diabetes* **30**, Suppl. 2, 76–81.

Schonfeld, G., Birge, C., Miller, J.P. et al (1974). Apolipoprotein B levels and altered lipoprotein composition in diabetes. *Diabetes* **23**, 827–834.

Sosenko, J.M., Breslow, J.L., Miettinen, O.S. et al (1980). Hyperglycaemia and plasma lipid levels. A prospective study of young insulin dependent diabetic patients. *New Engl. J. Med.* **302**, 650–654.

Stamler, R. and Stamler, J. (1979). Asymptomatic hyperglycaemia and coronary heart disease. A series of papers by the International Collaborative Group, based on studies on fifteen populations. *J. Chronic Dis.* **32**, 683–691.

Stamler, R., Stamler, J., Lindberg, H.A. et al (1979 a). Asymptomatic hyperglycemia and coronary heart disease in middle-aged men in two employed populations in Chicago. *J. Chronic Dis.* **32**, 805–815.

Stamler, R., Stamler, J., Schoenberger, J.A. et al (1979 b). Relationship of glucose tolerance to prevalence of ECG abnormalities and to 5-year mortality from cardiovascular disease: findings of the Chicago heart association detection project in industry. *J. Chronic Dis.* **32**, 817–828.

Steiner, G. (1981). Diabetes and atherosclerosis: an overview. *Diabetes* **30**, Suppl. 2, 1–7.

Sternby, N.H. (1968). Atherosclerosis in a defined population. An autopsy survey in Malmo, Sweden. *Acta Pathol. Microbiol. Scand.* Suppl. 194, 5–226.

Stocks, P. (1944). Diabetes mortality in 1861–1942 and some of the factors affecting it. *J. Hyg.* **43**, 242–247.

Stout, R.W. (1981). The role of insulin in atherosclerosis in diabetics and non-diabetics: a review. *Diabetes* **30**, Suppl. 2, 54–59.

Strandness, D.E., Priest, R.E. and Gibbons, G.E.

(1964). Combined clinical and pathological study of diabetic and non-diabetic peripheral arterial disease. *Diabetes* **13**, 366–372.

Tamborlane, W.V., Sherwin, R.S., Genel, M. et al (1979). Restoration of normal lipid and aminoacid metabolism in diabetic patients treated with a portable infusion pump. *Lancet* **i**, 1258–1261.

Taskinen, M.-R., Nikkila, E.A., Kuusi, T. et al (1982). Lipoprotein lipase activity and serum lipoproteins in untreated type 2 (insulin independent) diabetes associated with obesity. *Diabetologia* **22**, 46–50.

Taylor, K.G., Wright, A.D., Carter, T.J.N. et al (1981). High density lipoprotein cholesterol and apolipoprotein A-I levels at diagnosis in patients with non-insulin-dependent diabetes. *Diabetologia* **20**, 535–539.

University Group Diabetes Program (1970). A study of the effects of hypoglycaemic agents on vascular complications in patients with adult-onset diabetes. I: Design, methods and baseline results; II: Mortality results. *Diabetes* **19**, Suppl. 2, 747–830.

University Group Diabetes Program (1975). A study of the effects of hypoglycaemic agents on vascular complications in patients with adult-onset diabetes. V: Evaluation of phenformin therapy. *Diabetes* **24**, Suppl. 1, 65–184.

Verska, J.J. and Walker, W.J. (1975). Aortocoronary bypass in the diabetic patient. *Am. J. Cardiol.* **35**, 774–777.

Vigorita, V.J., Moore, G.W. and Hutchins, G.M. (1980). Absence of correlation between coronary arterial atherosclerosis and severity or duration of diabetes mellitus of adult onset. *Am. J. Cardiol.* **46**, 535–542.

Waller, B.F., Palumbo, P.J., Lie, J.T. et al (1980). Status of the coronary arteries at necropsy in diabetes mellitus with onset after age 30 years. Analysis of 229 diabetic patients with and without clinical evidence of coronary heart disease and comparison to 183 control subjects. *Am. J. Med.* **69**, 498–506.

Warren, S., Le Compte, P.M. and Legg, M.A. (1966). *The Pathology of Diabetes Mellitus.* Philadelphia, Lea & Febiger, 4th edn, p. 186.

Weaver, J.A., Bhatia, S.K., Boyle, D. et al (1970). Cardiovascular state of newly discovered diabetic women. *Br. Med. J.* **1**, 783–786.

Welborn, T.A. (1985). Macrovascular disease in Caucasoid diabetic patients. *Diabetologia,* **28**, 385–386.

Welborn, T.A., Knuiman, M., McCann, V. et al (1984). Clinical macrovascular disease in Caucasoid diabetic subjects; logistic regression analysis of risk variables. *Diabetologia* **27**, 568–573.

Welborn, T.A. and Wearne, K. (1979). Coronary heart disease incidence and cardiovascular mortality in Busselton with reference to glucose and insulin concentrations. *Diabetes Care* **2**, 154–160.

West, K.M. (1974). Diabetes in American Indians and other native populations of the New World. *Diabetes* **23**, 841–855.

West, K.M. (1978 a). *Epidemiology of Diabetes and its Vascular Lesions,* New York, Elsevier, pp. 172–176.

West, K.M. (1978 b). *Epidemiology of Diabetes and its Vascular Lesions,* New York, Elsevier, pp. 357–360.

West, K.M. (1978 c) *Epidemiology of Diabetes and its Vascular Lesions,* New York, Elsevier, pp. 389–402.

West, K.M. and Kalbfleisch, J.M. (1970). Diabetes in Central America. *Diabetes* **19**, pp. 656–663.

Westlund, K. (1969). *Mortality of Diabetics.* Life Insurance Companies' Institute for Medical Statistics at the Oslo City Hospitals, Report No. 13.

Xiaoren, P., Xuanhe, Z., Xiaofu, T. et al (1981). Diabetic complications. *Chin. Med. J.* **7**, 413–418.

Zdanov, V.S. and Vihert, A.M. (1976). Atherosclerosis and diabetes mellitus. *Bull. W.H.O.* **53**, 547–553.

Zimmet, P. (1979). Epidemiology of diabetes and its macrovascular manifestations in Pacific populations: the medical effects of social progress. *Diabetes Care* **2**, 144–153.

Chapter Two

Heart Disease and Diabetes Mellitus

R.D.S. Watson and S. Waldron

Dr Robert Watson qualified from Birmingham University in 1973 and trained in general medicine in Cardiff. As a Research Fellow in Cardiovascular Medicine in the University of Birmingham, he became interested in cardiovascular reflexes and blood pressure control in hypertension. He then spent a year at the Baker Medical Research Institute, Melbourne, studying biochemical methods of measuring sympathetic activity. In 1980 he was appointed Lecturer in Cardiovascular Medicine, University of Birmingham and Consultant Cardiologist in 1983.

Dr Sean Waldron qualified from University College, Galway in 1978 and completed his early training in Ireland. He came to England in 1984 and is researching cardiovascular aspects of diabetic autonomic neuropathy at Dudley Road Hospital, Birmingham.

Coronary Artery Disease

Diabetes with coronary artery disease may present with sudden death, acute myocardial infarction or angina pectoris; less frequently, patients present with left ventricular failure without clear evidence of previous myocardial infarction (Soler et al, 1975).

Diagnosis of Coronary Artery Disease

Diagnosis of CAD is based on the history and electrocardiographic (ECG) findings. A previous history of prolonged chest pain associated with pathological Q waves makes a diagnosis of previous acute myocardial infarction almost certain (rarely patients with hypertrophic cardiomyopathy have pathological Q waves not due to

coronary artery disease). Exercise-induced chest pain is likely to be ischaemic providing the possibility of a musculoskeletal origin is considered and excluded. Confounding factors which may cause ST/T wave changes include drugs (digoxin, psychotropic drugs), electrolyte changes especially hypokalaemia, hyperventilation, sympathetic stimulation (Taggart et al, 1979), and the mitral valve prolapse syndrome which may cause inferolateral ST depression or T inversion at rest or on exercise (Bisset et al, 1980). Glucose ingestion may produce ST depression or T-wave inversion; amongst 35 subjects with a high prevalence of cardiovascular risk factors, a previously normal fasting electrocardiogram became abnormal one hour after ingestion of a 75-g glucose drink in 11 subjects (Riley et al, 1972). In young diabetics, resting electrocardiographic changes are not increased in frequency (Karlefors, 1966). Amongst 18 000 middle-aged civil servants screened in the Whitehall study (Fuller et al, 1980), ECG changes were slightly more common in subjects with diabetes or glucose intolerance compared to euglycaemic subjects: ST depression (3 v. 1 per cent), left bundle block (1 v. 0.5 per cent) and T inversion (6 v. 4 per cent). In the diabetic subject, therefore, the findings of ST depression or T inversion on the resting ECG should be viewed with suspicion but are insufficient on their own to make a firm diagnosis of ischaemic heart disease.

Exercise testing

Exercise testing provides both diagnostic and prognostic information in the patient with symptoms suggestive of cardiac ischaemia. Its value in diagnosis depends importantly on the prevalence of coronary artery disease in the population studied. Thus, in middle-aged men with exertional chest pain, exercise-induced ST depression ($>$ 1 mm) confirms the clinical diagnosis of ischaemic heart disease with a high degree of confidence; a negative test in such a patient does not exclude ischaemia. On the other hand, amongst patients with a low prevalence of ischaemic heart disease (for example young women with atypical chest pain) a positive test occurs commonly in the absence of ischaemic heart disease (false positive test). The diagnostic sensitivity and specificity of exercise testing have not been reported in a diabetic population.

The exercise test has a valuable prognostic role. Patients with severe multivessel coronary artery disease may have mild or infrequent angina; exercise testing provides objective assessment of coronary vascular reserve. During exercise, development of chest pain or ST segment depression at a low work load, failure to achieve a heart rate of $>$ 120 beats/minute or an increase of systolic blood pressure of $>$ 20 mm Hg are associated with a high risk of later death or myocardial infarction (McNeer et al, 1978).

Karlefors (1966) performed exercise tests on 84 male diabetics (age 17–44 years) most of whom were insulin-dependent. Patients were free of clinical evidence of ischaemic heart disease and were compared to 76 healthy non-diabetic controls carefully matched for age. At four minutes after exercise, ST and T wave changes were observed more commonly amongst diabetics, the frequency increasing with duration of disease and prevalence of retinopathy. After an interval of 10 years, 71 of the original 84 diabetics were retested, together with half of the original controls (Persson, 1977). New resting ECG changes had developed in 17 per cent of diabetics (compared to 6 per cent of controls), and after exercise half the diabetics had ST/T wave changes compared to one-quarter of the controls. Of the 29 diabetics with abnormal ECGs originally studied in 1966, 31 per cent had sustained probable myocardial infarction compared to only 5 per cent of diabetics with normal ECG responses to exercise. During the 10-year period, amongst the diabetics, six deaths were attributed to myocardial infarction, two patients had had clinically diagnosed myocardial infarction and four had developed new electrocardiographic evidence of myocardial infarction; in contrast only one of the 46 controls had signs suggestive of myocardial infarction. This study suggests that nine of the 12 myocardial infarctions which developed in the diabetics during the 10-year follow-up were predicted from abnormal exercise test response at entry. These extremely important observations have major implications for detection and prevention of coronary heart disease in diabetics. However, these diabetics had a very high prevalence of smoking and the electrocardiograms appear to have been reclassified during the 10-year follow-up; furthermore, the study focussed on ischaemic changes occurring at four minutes after exercise rather than during maximal exercise. For these reasons, confirmation of these results seems desirable.

Radionuclide studies

These methods have a useful role in the diagnosis of ischaemic heart disease; however, their role in diagnosis in diabetics has not been fully evaluated.

After intravenous injection, thallium-201 is distributed with coronary blood flow and taken up by adequately perfused myocardium. Injection during exercise followed by scintigraphy shortly afterwards usually reveals perfusion defects in patients with severe proximal coronary stenosis. Repeat scintigraphy several hours later may show that the defect has disappeared, indicating that reversible exercise-induced ischaemia was originally present; a persisting defect after redistribution usually indicates myocardial scar as a result of previous infarction.

Thallium-201 scans performed in 12 middle-aged male diabetics free of clinical evidence of ischaemic heart disease revealed perfusion defects in five patients, four irreversible and one reversible. Only one of 12 healthy non-diabetic controls demonstrated a reversible defect (Abenavoli et al, 1981). These studies may indicate a high prevalence of clinically undetected coronary artery disease in diabetics. Alternatively, focal myocardial fibrosis may have been responsible. In patients with systemic lupus erythematosus, in whom vasculitis is an important complication, similar thallium defects were observed in 38 per cent of patients (Hosenpud et al, 1984). The significance of these findings will remain uncertain until further studies correlating thallium defects with coronary angiographic findings in diabetics have been performed. Therefore, thallium scans must be interpreted with caution in diabetic patients.

Technetium ventriculography is useful in the diagnosis of ischaemic heart disease, the development of localised areas of asynergy or a fall in ejection fraction during exercise indicating myocardial ischaemia. However, a high prevalence of abnormal responses has been reported in diabetic patients free of clinical evidence of ischaemic heart disease, suggesting that the diagnostic value of technetium ventriculography is limited in diabetics (Vered et al, 1984) (see below).

Coronary angiography

Choice of patients for coronary angiography is determined partly by the role of surgery. Patients with angina which restricts life-style despite medical treatment are potential candidates for coronary artery bypass grafting (CABG); others with less severe symptoms in whom exercise testing suggests severe multivessel coronary disease may also be considered, particularly those with electrocardiographic evidence of severe ischaemia at low work-load; patients with angina following myocardial infarction are also at increased risk and may benefit from surgery. Patients with angina, left ventricular failure or recurrent ventricular tachyarrhythmias associated with ventricular aneurysm are candidates for left ventricular aneurysmectomy; grafting of stenosed vessels supplying viable myocardium is performed at the same time so that preoperative coronary angiography is essential in these patients. Coronary angiography carries a risk of death of less than 0.1 per cent; patients with severe left ventricular dysfunction and severe multivessel coronary disease are at greatest risk. Before investigation, the presence of atheroma in lower limb vessels should be carefully assessed in the diabetic; in those with lower limb ischaemia, the femoral route should be avoided in favour of the brachial route.

The predisposition of the diabetic to atheroma has led to the belief that diffuse coronary artery disease may make these patients unsuitable for CABG. A retrospective study of angiographic findings in 37 diabetics who were matched for age, sex, smoking, hypertension and hyperlipidaemia with 79 non-diabetic controls does not support this belief (Dortimer et al, 1978). Significant stenoses were found in more vessels in diabetics than controls, double or triple vessel disease being present in three-quarters of diabetics compared to half the controls. However, the number of vessels which were diffusely diseased was similar, 22 per cent in diabetics compared to 28 per cent in controls. Diffuse disease sufficient to preclude successful revascularisation affected 4 per cent of diabetic vessels and 6 per cent of control vessels. Thus, diabetic coronary arteries do not seem to be more likely to develop diffuse disease sufficient to prevent successful CABG.

Heparin is usually administered before coronary angiography and reversed by protamine at completion. A high incidence of allergic reactions to protamine following angiography has been reported amongst diabetics (Stewart et al, 1984). Since haemostasis can usually be achieved without heparin reversal, protamine administration should usually be avoided. Successful CABG surgery has been reported in two patients with protamine allergy; heparin was reversed by platelet concentrates instead of protamine at completion of surgery (Walker et al, 1984).

The role of surgery

Table 2.1 presents the results of CABG from diabetic patients undergoing surgery during the 1970s; improvements in surgical technique and myocardial preservation during the last decade may be expected to result in more favourable mortality rates. Compared to non-diabetics, mortality rates in diabetics were consistently higher and ranged from 4 to 11 per cent; in the largest series reported (Johnson et al, 1982) 4.7 per cent mortality was observed amongst 190 diabetics with good left ventricular function. Morbidity was also greater, mainly due to sepsis, stroke and renal impairment. Surgery was successful in achieving a substantial improvement in symptoms in at least three-quarters of patients; long-term survival was similar to that observed in operated non-diabetics, with 90 per cent five-year survival in diabetics with good left venticular function and 57 per cent in diabetics with poor left ventricular function (66 per cent in non-diabetic controls) (Johnson et al, 1982).

These results suggest that the results and risks of CABG are acceptable in diabetics who have troublesome angina despite medical treatment with two or three anti-anginal drugs.

Results of left ventricular aneurysmectomy have not been reported in diabetics. However, the operation is known to carry a greater mortality than CABG alone; success depends critically upon the function of the left ventricle remaining after aneurysm resection. Two-dimensional echocardiography and technetium ventriculography may provide useful non-invasive inform-

Table 2.1 Summary of surgical mortality and morbidity in diabetic patients undergoing coronary artery bypass grafting

Author	Date of surgery	No. of Diabetics	In-hospital mortality (%)		Morbidity (%)
			DM	*Controls*	
Johnson et al (1982)	1971–77	261	9.2	3.1	11.6
			Good LV 4.7	1.6	(Stroke, bleeding
			Poor LV 15.7	8.6	infection)
Engelman et al (1976)	1972	24	4.0	1.0 (Non-hypertensive, non-diabetic controls)	8.0 (Low cardiac output, renal impairment)
Verska & Walker (1975)	1971–73	35	11.0	4.0	15 complications in 35 patients (cf. 21 complications in 77 non-diabetics)
Chychota et al (1973)	1966–71	13	8.0	5.0	11.0 (excess infection)

DM, Diabetes mellitus.

ation concerning left ventricular function before invasive angiography and surgery. Since the operation has not been demonstrated to improve long-term outcome in patients with few or no symptoms, it should probably be considered only in patients with symptoms of at least moderate severity after determined efforts at medical treatment.

Surgical risks are increased in the presence of cerebrovascular disease, which should be regarded as a relative contraindication. In some centres, patients with a carotid bruit undergo carotid angiography and endarterectomy before CABG. Other relative contraindications to surgery include severe peripheral vascular disease which limits physical activity, since further arterial surgery may be necessary following CABG, and poor left ventricular function (ejection fraction <30 per cent), since this is associated with increased surgical mortality.

Should CABG be considered in patients with less severe angina? At present, no follow-up studies are available which indicate the likely five-year mortality in medically treated diabetics with mild symptoms of ischaemic heart disease. Such information is essential in order to assess the possible value of early surgery in diabetics. Two trials performed in non-diabetics have yielded conflicting results. A European multi-centre trial (European Coronary Surgery Study Group, 1982) indicated favourable improvement in outcome following early surgery in patients with double or triple vessel coronary disease involving the proximal left anterior descending coronary artery. No benefit was observed in the Coronary Artery Surgery Study (CASS) CASS Principal Investigators and their Associates, 1983), regardless of the number of vessels diseased. The important difference between the trials lay in the mortality in the medically treated groups which was low (8 per cent at five years) in CASS and substantially higher (16 per cent at five years) in the European study. At present it seems wise to restrict CABG to diabetics with moderately severe symptoms, particularly in view of their slightly increased surgical mortality.

Role of Coronary Angioplasty

The value of coronary angioplasty is an area of intense research, and it is possible that the technique may become established in unstable angina and acute myocardial infarction. At present, patients with stable angina with proximal discrete non-calcified stenoses in one or two coronary arteries are considered ideal. The procedure carries a small risk of death (about 1 per cent) or myocardial infarction (5–10 per cent) and some patients require urgent CABG (about 6 per cent) (Willman, 1985). Since these patients with single- or double-vessel disease would be considered to be at low risk with medical treatment, at present the procedure should be reserved for patients with moderately troublesome angina or other evidence of increased risk (e.g., severe ST depression at low work-load). In non-diabetics the restenosis rate is about 25 per cent at six months, these patients often undergoing repeat dilatation at low risk; in a small series restenosis occurred in 75 per cent of 12 diabetic patients (Margolis et al, 1984). Further studies are essential to determine whether diabetics are at increased risks of restenosis and to clarify the role of angioplasty in patients with relative contra-indications to CABG (e.g., cerebrovascular disease and poor left ventricular function).

Medical Treatment

Nitrates, β-receptor antagonists and calcium-channel antagonists provide the mainstay of medical treatment in patients with ischaemic heart disease. Many physicians accept the evidence from several trials which indicate a significant advantage of β-receptor antagonists in prevention of sudden death and reinfarction during the first one or two years following acute myocardial infarction (Chamberlain, 1983; Baber et al, 1984). However, these observations cannot neccessarily be extrapolated to patients with stable angina free of recent infarction. Similarly, evidence that nitrates or calcium-channel antagonists prevent death or infarction in patients with angina is lacking. Therefore, the choice of drugs must be determined by the severity of symptoms, tolerance of specific side-effects, likelihood of adverse effects and presence of coexisting disease.

Nitrates

All patients with angina should receive careful instruction, preferably written, in the use of sublingual glyceryl trinitrate (GTN) or a suitable alternative (e.g., GTN spray or chewable isosorbide dinitrate). These drugs are particularly effective in the small group of patients with variant or Prinzmetal angina associated with transient ST segment elevation which is usually due to coronary artery spasm (often associated with fixed coronary stenosis). Long-acting nitrates (e.g., isosorbide dinitrate) are effective antianginal agents with a duration of action of up to eight hours; careful titration to maximally effective dose is essential. Patients should be warned of headache which can be minimised by titration from low doses; nevertheless, many patients find this symptom intolerable. Isosorbide mononitrate has a theoretical advantage of not being subject to variable first-pass metabolism and providing more predictable plasma levels; however, clinical advantages have not been convincingly demonstrated. Cutaneous preparations may simplify management for patients requiring many other tablets by mouth, but they are expensive and their efficacy and particularly their claimed long duration of action have been questioned recently (Abrams, 1984). Nitrates probably exert their major antianginal effect by reducing left ventricular filling pressure, wall stress and oxygen requirements; in contrast to β-receptor antagonists and calcium-channel antagonists they have no negative inotropic effects and therefore are particularly useful in patients with left ventricular dysfunction. They should be used cautiously in patients with diabetic autonomic neuropathy since baroreflex dysfunction may impair buffering of blood pressure and cause hypotension.

ß-Adrenoceptor antagonists

The proven efficacy of these drugs in the treatment of angina is mainly a consequence of antagonism of cardiac β_1 receptors leading to blunted chronotropic and inotropic responses to sympathetic stimulation during exercise. Additional blockade of β_2 receptors is unlikely to be helpful in diabetics since this may unmask or exacerbate symptoms of peripheral vascular disease due to blunting of β_2-receptor-mediated vasodilatation. Additionally, β_2-receptor blockade may exaggerate the pressor response to insulin-induced hypoglycaemia and may lead to profound reflex bradycardia (Lloyd-Mostyn & Oram, 1975; Lager et al, 1979); furthermore, delayed recovery of blood glucose levels following hypoglycaemia is more likely in patients treated with non-selective β-adrenoceptor antagonists (Deacon & Barnett, 1976; Deacon et al, 1977; Lager et al, 1979). For these reasons, many physicians prefer to treat diabetics, particularly type I diabetics, with drugs which are relatively specific for β_1 receptors, for example, atenolol, metoprolol. Since these drugs are effective antihypertensive drugs, they are particularly useful in the hypertensive diabetic with angina.

Reversible airways obstruction and peripheral vascular disease are major contraindications to these drugs. In patients with left ventricular impairment causing breathlessness, cardiomegaly or a third heart sound, β-adrenoceptor antagonists should be used with great caution: drugs with vasodilator properties such as calcium antagonists (e.g., nifedipine) or nitrates are preferable.

β-Adrenoceptor antagonists may cause deterioration of blood glucose control. Increases of blood glucose of 1–2 mmol/l occur commonly (Wright et al, 1979), but greater increases are infrequent unless patients are treated concurrently with a thiazide diuretic (Dornhorst et al, 1985). If combination of β-adrenoceptor antagonist and diuretic is essential, a loop diuretic such as furosemide or bumetanide may be preferable to a thiazide.

Despite these possible disadvantages, the

physician should not be deterred from using selective β-adrenoceptor antagonists in diabetics since they have an important therapeutic role. However, careful patient selection is essential and more frequent measurement of blood glucose levels is wise in the weeks following introduction.

Calcium-channel antagonists

The introduction of calcium-channel antagonists has been a major advance in cardiovascular therapy during the last decade. Currently, three drugs, diltiazem, nifedipine and verapamil, are in use in the UK; their individual haemodynamic effects and side-effects differ considerably. All cause relaxation of vascular smooth muscle. The sinus and atrioventricular (AV) nodes are dependent on membrane calcium fluxes, and verapamil and diltiazem may cause bradycardia and prolongation of atrioventricular conduction. These electrophysiological effects are a major advantage in patients with supraventricular tachyarrhythmia (e.g., atrioventricular nodal reciprocating tachycardia, atrial flutter and fibrillation) in which verapamil has an established role; in patients with sinus node or atrioventricular node disease, both diltiazem and verapamil should be avoided. Nifedipine, however, has negligible electrophysiological effects. Potential direct negative inotropic effects of these drugs tend to be offset by simultaneous vasodilatation and, in general, nifedipine is well tolerated in patients with impaired left ventricular function; however, diltiazem and verapamil should be used cautiously in patients with significant left ventricular dysfunction.

Side-effects with nifedipine and diltiazem are related to their potent vasodilating effects leading to palpitation, headache, flushing and oedema; rarely, hypotension and tachycardia following nifedipine have caused exacerbation of angina. Verapamil commonly causes constipation and patients should be warned of the need to increase dietary fibre. Plasma digoxin levels increase with concurrent verapamil treatment and digoxin doses should therefore be reduced or

plasma concentrations checked within seven days (Klein et al, 1982).

In vitro, calcium-channel antagonists inhibit insulin release from islet cells. In intact man, however, the influence of these drugs on glucose tolerance is uncertain. Nifedipine (20 mg three times a day for three days) was reported to increase blood glucose and inhibit insulin responses during oral glucose tolerance tests (100 g) in normal subjects (Charles et al, 1981); similarly, Giugliano et al (1980) observed impaired glucose tolerance and reduced insulin responses in chemical diabetics after nifedipine (10 mg three times a day for 10 days). Precipitation of clinical diabetes has been described in case reports of five hypertensives treated with nifedipine (Bhatnagar et al, 1984; Zezulka et al, 1984); a small but significant increase in random blood glucose (0.3 mmol) was reported (Zezulka et al, 1984) after treatment of hypertensive non-diabetics mostly receiving other antihypertensive drugs. On the other hand, several authors have reported no significant change in glucose tolerance and insulin release after treatment of normal subjects and Type 2 diabetics with nifedipine (Donnelly and Harrower, 1980; Greenwood, 1982; Jaffe et al, 1983). Evidence concerning verapamil is also conflicting: improved glucose tolerance and unchanged insulin responses were observed in non-obese Type II diabetics after intravenous or oral verapamil treatment (Rojdmark and Andersson, 1984); in non-diabetic subjects, intravenous verapamil did not alter hepatic vein glucose and insulin responses to oral glucose. It was concluded that verapamil was unlikely to inhibit pancreatic insulin release but may facilitate hepatic uptake of glucose (Rojdmark and Andersson, 1984). After 10 days oral verapamil treatment, unchanged glucose and insulin responses to oral glucose were observed in non-diabetics (Giugliano et al, 1981); however, a small decrease in insulin response to small (5 g) but not larger (20 g) intravenous glucose pulses was observed in non-diabetics after intravenous verapamil; insulin and glucagon responses to arginine were also impaired. Similarly, intravenous verapamil impaired insulin responses in normal subjects following glucose, glucagon and glibenclamide administration (Giugliano et al, 1981). These studies suggest that insulin responses to a variety of stimuli may be impaired by calcium-channel antagonists but the clinical relevance of this remains uncertain. Unfortunately, most of the studies have been conducted in very small numbers of subjects over short periods. Long-term studies in normal subjects and Types 1 and 2 diabetics are needed in order to assess the possible diabetogenic effects of calcium-channel antagonists. In the meantime, clinicians must be aware of the possibility of deterioration in glucose tolerance and should check blood glucose levels after initiation of treatment with calcium-channel antagonists.

Choice of drugs

Formal comparisons of the efficacy of these drugs in diabetic patients have not been reported. In patients with occasional angina, a supply of nitrates may be all that is required. Calcium-channel antagonists or nitrates are preferable in patients with airways disease, peripheral vascular disease or left ventricular impairment; these drugs may be safely combined. β-Adrenoceptor antagonists or calcium-channel antagonists are preferable in hypertensive patients. Many patients with troublesome angina may require two or three drugs in combination. Calcium-channel antagonists, such as nifedipine and possibly diltiazem, may be safely combined with β-adrenoceptor antagonists. The use of verapamil with a β-adrenoceptor antagonist may lead to an increased risk of negative inotropic and chronotropic effects leading to conduction disorders and heart failure; their combined use should be considered only under careful medical supervision.

Acute Myocardial Infarction in Diabetics

Acute myocardial infarction is a major complication of diabetes which carries a high mortality (Table 2.2). In-hospital mortality was approximately doubled in three of four studies which described acute infarction in diabetics (Harrower

Table 2.2 Mortality rates in diabetic patients following acute myocardial infarction

Author	Period of study	Duration of follow-up (months)	Mortality in diabetic patients (%)	Mortality in controls (%)
Partamian & Bradley (1965)	1954–58	2	38 (first MI)	—
		60	62 (first MI)	—
		2	55 (2nd or subsequent MI)	—
		60	75 (2nd or subsequent MI)	—
Soler et al (1975)	1967–73	1	40	—
		12	51	—
Gwilt et al (1984a)	1967–81	In-hospital	33	17.4
Harrower & Clarke (1976)	1968–73	In-hospital	24	19
Tansey et al (1977)	1972–74	In-hospital	28	14
Jaffe et al (1984)	1975	12	33	22
Czyzk et al (1980)	1980	In-hospital	36	18
Smith et al (1984)		12	30 (survivors of CCU)	8

MI, Myocardial infarct; CCU, Coronary Care Unit.

& Clark, 1976; Tansey et al, 1977; Czyzk et al, 1980; Gwilt et al, 1984a); increased risk continued during the first one to two years following infarction (Jaffe et al, 1984; Smith et al, 1984).

The high early mortality is largely due to an increased risk of pump failure; ventricular arrhythmias after the coronary care phase may also contribute significantly (Harrower & Clarke, 1976). Amongst 353 diabetics with infarction. Gwilt and colleagues (1984a) reported 118 deaths (33 per cent) in hospital; 93 per cent of deaths were due to cardiac failure. In two smaller studies, pump failure accounted for 52 per cent (Tansey et al, 1977) and 75 per cent (Harrower & Clarke, 1976) of in-hospital deaths. Jaffe et al (1984) observed an increased risk of pulmonary congestion amongst diabetics with infarction (31 per cent compared to 16 per cent in controls); amongst diabetics with previous infarction the risk was more clearly accentuated (50 per cent compared to 16 per cent in controls).

Many factors in the diabetic might lead to an increased risk of haemodynamic complications. Presentation with little or no chest pain occurs more commonly (Partamian & Bradley, 1965), and this may lead to delay in diagnosis and treatment. In a large study of 285 diabetics with infarction, presenting symptoms were heart failure (13 per cent), uncontrolled diabetes (7 per cent), vomiting (5 per cent), collapse (3 per cent), confusion (2 per cent) and stroke (2 per cent); in this study one-third of patients were admitted to the general medical wards rather than the coronary care unit due to difficulty in recognising the nature of the presenting illness (Soler et al, 1975). It is unlikely that the presenting myocardial infarction is larger in diabetics than controls since serial measurements of cardiac enzyme release as an index of infarct size have not shown marked differences (Gwilt et al, 1984 b). However, it is possible that more severe coronary artery disease is present in diabetics with infarction, since in one study angina was present more frequently both before and after infarction (Smith et al, 1984); furthermore, in a large necropsy study, left main coronary stenosis was found more commonly in diabetics

who died (mainly of acute coronary events) compared to non-diabetic coronary deaths (Waller et al, 1980). Acute metabolic disturbance is a common complication of infarction in diabetics. Attempts to achieve excellent diabetic control using intravenous insulin infusion during the acute phase have not resulted in a clear-cut reduction in mortality: amongst 65 diabetics, including 55 previously treated with oral hypoglycaemic drugs or insulin, in-hospital mortality was unchanged (Gwilt et al, 1984a); on the other hand, in a small study of 39 patients previously treated with oral hypoglycaemic agents or insulin, treatment with intravenous insulin was associated with a decrease in mortality from 48 per cent (10 of 21 patients) to 11 per cent (two of 18 patients) (Clark et al, 1985).

Several observations suggest that the high mortality following acute infarction in diabetics may be related to the increased frequency of previously unrecognised infarction in these patients. In the Framingham survey, silent infarction was detected during follow-up in 39 per cent of diabetics compared to 22 per cent of matched controls (Garcia et al, 1974). Necropsy examination revealed healed transmural infarction in 89 per cent of diabetics who died of coronary heart disease compared to 48 per cent of non-diabetics; amongst diabetics free of clinical evidence of heart disease before death, healed scars were present in 22 per cent (Waller et al, 1980). Clinically healthy diabetics had a high frequency of abnormal thallium-201 scintigrams at rest (four of 16 subjects), suggestive of previous silent infarction (Abenavoli et al, 1981). Furthermore, persistently positive technetium pyrophosphate myocardial scintigrams were reported more commonly (62 per cent) following acute myocardial infarction in diabetics compared to non-diabetics (Nicod et al, 1982); these patients had a higher complication rate than those without persistently positive scans. Histological examination often revealed scar intermixed with acute and chronic cellular injury, and these persistently positive scans may therefore reflect acute infarction at the site of previous ischaemic fibrosis.

Finally, autonomic neuropathy may impair sympathetically mediated inotropic responses during acute infarction. However, since responses to autonomic function tests are frequently altered following infarction, the role of autonomic neuropathy in determining outcome from acute infarction must await the results of a prospective study.

It is difficult to ascertain from published series whether pump failure in diabetics is established early or occurs as a late complication, for example following infarct extension or arrhythmias; in one study, approximately half the deaths occurred after transfer from the coronary care unit (Soler et al, 1974). The role of acute intervention with β-adrenoceptor antagonists in preventing complications in acute myocardial infarction is uncertain. Previously published studies in non-diabetics have shown no consistent benefit of acute treatment (Anon, 1982; Yusuf et al, 1985). Although intravenous followed by oral treatment with metoprolol was reported to reduce mortality at three months (Hjalmarson et al, 1981), a large multicentre trial using identical treatment revealed a non-significant reduction in mortality of 13 per cent at 15 days (MIAMI Trial Research Group, 1985). In this study, diabetics constituted 7 per cent of the trial population; retrospective analysis demonstrated a significant ($P<0.05$) reduction of 15-day mortality in diabetics receiving active treatment (11 deaths in 192 patients, 5.7 per cent) compared to those receiving placebo (25 deaths in 221 patients, 11.3 per cent). Although retrospective subgroup analysis requires cautious interpretation, these observations suggest the possibility of an important role for β-adrenoceptor antagonists in diabetics with acute myocardial infarction; further studies will be necessary to confirm these observations and to indicate the likely number of diabetics with infarction who are free of contraindications to drug treatment at admission to hospital.

A consistent reduction in long-term mortality has been demonstrated in several trials of β-adrenoceptor antagonist treatment initiated some days after acute myocardial infarction in non-diabetics. In the timolol trial in which treatment was started after an average interval of 10 days (Norwegian Multicentre Study Group, 1981), total mortality during a mean follow-up period of 17 months was significantly reduced from 15.5 per cent in placebo-treated patients to 10.3 per cent in those receiving timolol. Retrospective analysis revealed that in 46 diabetic patients allocated to placebo (Gundersen & Kjekshus, 1983), the total mortality was 30.5 per cent, confirming the increased risk among diabetic patients with infarction; in contrast, 53 diabetics allocated randomly to timolol treatment had a significantly lower mortality (11.3 per cent); a significant reduction in reinfarction rate was also observed (3.8 per cent v. 21.7 per cent). Thirty-four per cent of timolol-treated diabetics were withdrawn compared to 26 per cent of patients receiving placebo, suggesting that active treatment was infrequently responsible for side-effects. These results indicate that diabetics, like non-diabetics, should receive treatment with β-adrenoceptor antagonist drugs for one to two years following acute myocardial infarction, providing that patients are free of major contraindications to treatment.

Thrombolytic agents administered during the acute phase of myocardial infarction are currently undergoing extensive evaluation (Laffel & Braunwald, 1984). Reperfusion of the obstructed coronary artery subtending the infarct zone has been achieved in about three-quarters of patients using intracoronary streptokinase administered within six hours of onset of symptoms. Slightly lower success rates have been achieved using the intravenous route which has potentially major advantages including shorter delay time, lower cost and being less invasive. Recently, tissue type plasminogen activator has been used to produce clot lysis without a systemic lytic state. Most trials have failed to demonstrate a major reduction in mortality or improvement in global left ventricular function following thrombolytic treatment; final judgement must await the results of large trials using optimal therapeutic regimes administered soon after onset of symptoms; additionally, other procedures such as CABG or angioplasty may be necessary to prevent reocclusion of successfully recanalised arteries.

The Electrocardiogram and Conduction Disorders in Diabetes

A slightly increased prevalence of resting ST/T-wave changes and left bundle branch block in otherwise healthy diabetics has already been described (Fuller et al, 1980). Resting and exercise electrocardiograms should preferably be performed in the fasting state (>three hours postprandial) in view of the possible effects of glucose ingestion in causing transient ST/T-wave changes (Riley et al, 1972).

Twenty-four-hour electrocardiographic recording amongst healthy diabetics has revealed no excess of brady- or tachyarrhythmias. Diabetics with autonomic neuropathy have higher daytime heart rates and a reduced slowing of heart rate during sleep, reflecting impaired vagal function, when compared to diabetics free of autonomic neuropathy (Ewing et al, 1983).

Diabetics may be at increased risk of developing severe conduction disorders. Fairfax and Leatham (1975) reported that 9 per cent of patients undergoing permanent pacemaker implantation for complete heart block were diabetic (2 per cent Type 1, 7 per cent Type 2); in this population, vitiligo, hypothyroidism and pernicious anaemia were also more common suggesting a common autoimmune aetiology. In a German study (Hasslacher & Wahl, 1977), 23 per cent of patients undergoing permanent pacemaker implantation were longstanding diabetics with a further 18 per cent diagnosed at the time of implantation; the frequency of diabetes was similar in those paced for sinus node disease and atrioventricular block. Among 200 diabetics without overt diabetes, first-degree heart block was observed in 7 per cent and right bundle branch block in 6.5 per cent; these conduction disorders were significantly more common when compared to a hypertensive control group but no information concerning prevalence in healthy controls was given (Blandford & Burden, 1984).

Diabetics with symptoms of dizziness or syncope which could be due to arrhythmias should undergo investigation with a resting electrocardiogram, followed, if necessary, by a 24-hour ECG recording. If symptoms are infrequent, the patient may be provided with a small recorder which can pick up the electrocardiograph by placement on the chest and recording for 20–30 seconds during symptoms; the signal may be transmitted transtelephonically to a suitable receiver at the hospital for decoding. Permanent pacemaker implantation should be undertaken in symptomatic patients with complete heart block (persistent or intermittent). Mobitz Type 2 AV block, prolonged sinus pauses or severe bradycardia (<35–40 beats/minute). In patients with less severe bradycardias or intermittent Mobitz Type I (Wenkebach) block, efforts should be made to try to demonstrate that the conduction disorder occurs at the time of symptoms, since these rhythm disturbances may occur in healthy subjects. In asymptomatic patients, the incidental finding of a severe conduction disorder on the resting electrocardiogram, for example, bifascicular block with RBBB and left or right axis deviation, should not necessarily lead to prophylactic pacemaker insertion since the risk of progression to symptomatic complete heart block is low (Alpert & Flaker, 1984).

Specific Heart Muscle Disease in Diabetes Mellitus

Terminology

Cardiomyopathy is defined as "a disorder of heart muscle of unknown cause or association" (Goodwin, 1972). The term diabetic cardiomyopathy is therefore a misnomer. Disorders of heart muscle in diabetes mellitus should be referred to as diabetes mellitus specific heart muscle disease (HMD) or, more conveniently, diabetic HMD.

Epidemiological, morphological and clinical studies all point towards an increased prevalence of heart muscle disease in diabetes mellitus.

Epidemiological evidence

Follow-up of patients enrolled in the Framingham Survey (Garcia et al, 1974; Kannel & McGee, 1979) indicates a greatly increased risk of developing cardiovascular disease in diabetics. In male diabetics age-adjusted risk of developing cardiovascular disease or congestive heart failure was approximately doubled; in women, the impact of diabetes was even greater with a relative risk of 2.8 for cardiovascular disease and 5.4 for congestive heart failure. After allowance for the influence of other risk factors (e.g., hypertension, smoking, electrocardiographic changes at entry), the high risk persisted, particularly for women (relative adjusted risk 3.8 for development of congestive heart failure). Insulin-treated women appeared to be at particularly high risk. While the increased prevalence of ischaemic heart disease probably accounts for some of this increased risk, evidence from other sources suggests that diabetic HMD may be important.

Pathological studies

The concept of small-vessel disease as a cause of diabetic HMD developed from the observations of Blumenthal et al (1960) who described endothelial swelling and proliferation, occasionally progressing to obstruction, in intramural coronary arteries (diameter 70–150 μm) in approximately one-third of diabetics examined at postmortem. Similar findings have been confirmed by others (Hamby et al, 1974; Crall & Roberts, 1978; Zoneraich et al, 1980). Ledet later performed two careful quantitative studies in young and older diabetics (Ledet, 1968, 1976). Proliferative endothelial lesions sufficient to obstruct intramural coronary arteries were not observed. However, positive staining for periodic acid–Schiff (PAS) reagent was found more commonly in the tunica media in diabetics; in elderly diabetics the prevalence was 75 per cent and 60 per cent in small (20–60 μm) and medium (70–150 μm) vessels, respectively, compared to 35 per cent and 25 per cent respectively, in non-diabetics; amongst young diabetics the prevalence in small vessels was 75 per cent compared to 33 per cent in non-diabetics. Mucopolysaccharide deposition was not sufficient to reduce the luminal diameter and the number of affected vessels was not increased. The relatively sparse nature of these lesions suggests that an important obstructive angiopathy of small- and medium-sized vessels is unlikely in diabetic heart muscle disease; clinical studies in patients with left ventricular dysfunction not associated with significant obstruction of large- and medium-sized coronary arteries failed to demonstrate abnormal lactate metabolism during rapid atrial pacing (Regan et al, 1977), further suggesting that small-vessel disease does not lead to myocardial ischaemia.

Deposition of collagen material, often PAS positive, distributed around blood vessels and penetrating between muscle cells has been a consistent finding in diabetics dying with heart failure unrelated to large coronary vessel disease. (Rubler et al, 1972; Hamby et al, 1974; Ledet, 1976; Regan et al, 1977). The lesions of intramural vessels described above may reflect a generalised deposition of collagen material in the hearts of these patients. Regan observed interstitial deposition of PAS-positive material in dogs rendered diabetic by streptozotocin and in spontaneously diabetic dogs (Regan et al, 1974).

In a postmortem study of nine diabetics who died from non-ischaemic heart failure, Factor and co-workers (1980a) observed similar morphological abnormalities with interstitial fibrosis and extensive scar formation. These patients all had previous hypertension: when compared to non-diabetic hypertensives and non-hypertensive diabetics, the morphological changes in the hypertensive diabetics were much more extensive. Subsequent studies in rats made hypertensive by renal clipping and diabetic by streptozotocin led to very similar pathological changes (Fein et al, 1984); these authors emphasised that it is the combination of diabetes and hypertension which results in marked cardiac fibrosis, whereas diabetes or hypertension alone were much less damaging.

Recently, capillary microaneurysms have been demonstrated in myocardial capillaries in diabetics using silicone rubber injection at postmortem (Figure 2.1) (Factor et al, 1980b). These lesions were similar to those well recognised in the eye and the kidney in diabetics. Interstitial fibrosis was commonly seen in these hearts but, thus far, detailed studies relating the distribution of fibrosis with microaneurysms have not been reported. Further evidence of ultrastructural changes in diabetes has been demonstrated in myocardial biopsy material obtained from diabetics undergoing coronary artery surgery (Fischer et al, 1979). Increased thickening of capillary basal lamina membranes was demonstrated in the diabetics as previously observed in other tissues; of interest, patients with glucose intolerance without clinical diabetes had lamina thickness intermediate between

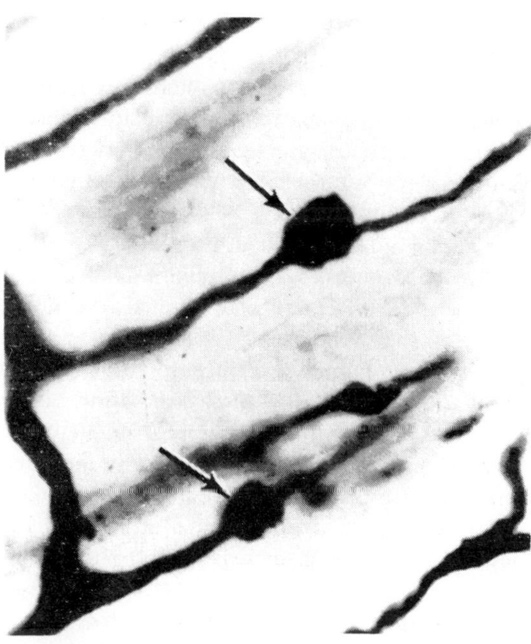

Figure 2.1 Photomicrograph of myocardium from a Type 1 diabetic patient reveals capillary loops with microaneurysms (arrows). The vessels have been perfused with a silicone rubber compound and magnified × 900. Reprinted by permission of the *New England Journal of Medicine* **302**, 386, 1980.

diabetics and controls. These ultrastructural changes may prove to be of considerable importance in the development of the interstitial fibrosis commonly observed in the failing diabetic myocardium.

Clinical studies

Systolic time intervals

This method allows non-invasive assessment of cardiac function derived from timing of electrical (electrocardiogram) and mechanical events (phonocardiogram and external carotid pulse). The total period of electrical and mechanical events during left ventricular systole is timed from the onset of the Q wave to the aortic component of the second heart sound (QS_2). This period is made up of two components: the pre-ejection period (PEP) (from onset of electrical activity to start of ejection) and the left ventricular ejection time (LVET) (from the upstroke to the incisura of the carotid pulse tracing)

$$PEP = QS_2 - LVET$$

After correction for heart rate, PEP and LVET provide reproducible measurements of left ventricular function. In left ventricular dysfunction of all types, PEP tends to increase and LVET to decrease. Thus, the ratio PEP/LVET provides a very sensitive, although non-specific, measure of cardiac function. A decrease in LVET is easily understood as a consequence of reduced velocity of ejection; an increase in PEP is attributed to a reduced rate of contraction of myocardial fibres during the isovolumic contraction time from mitral valve closure to onset of ejection into the aorta.

A number of studies in diabetics indicate that PEP is often prolonged and LVET shortened consistent with impaired LV function (Ahmed et al, 1975; Seneviratne, 1977; Zoneraich et al, 1977; Shapiro et al, 1981a; Uusitupa et al, 1983). Although these abnormalities appeared to be independent of the mode of treatment, it is possible that some of the changes may reflect poor diabetic control since Sykes et al (1977) observed improved systolic time intervals after treatment of previously untreated diabetics with oral hypoglycaemic agents; furthermore, Uusitupa et al (1983) observed that values improved in those patients treated with diet who achieved a fall of blood glucose of greater than 3 mmol/l. However, abnormal systolic time intervals appear to become more common in patients in the presence of diabetic microvascular complications. In three studies which excluded patients with these complications, systolic time intervals were found to be similar to normal controls (Rubler et al, 1978; Friedman et al, 1982; Posner et al, 1983). On the other hand, Seneviratne (1977) observed abnormal systolic time intervals only in patients with microvascular complications; Shapiro and colleagues (1981b) confirmed that recently diagnosed diabetics and those free from microangiopathy usually had normal values, whereas patients with severe microangiopathy frequently had abnormal values. These studies therefore provide consistent evidence that a non-specific abnormality of left ventricular function commonly accompanies the presence of diabetic microangiopathic disease in other organs.

Echocardiography

Ultrasound examination of the heart is a reproducible non-invasive method which allows measurement of cardiac chamber size as well as timing of intracardiac events such as mitral valve opening and closure. M mode echocardiography allows measurement of cardiac chamber size in one axis only; therefore deductions about chamber volumes are very limited. Thus far, no studies using two-dimensional echocardiography in diabetics have been reported. A major limitation of the method is the practical difficulty of obtaining high-quality echocardiograms suitable for accurate measurement, especially in the obese and elderly. Ideally, measurements of left ventricular dimension should be made over a number of cardiac cycles by an observer who is unaware of the patient's clinical status. In practice, few studies have used a truly blind independent observer.

Two studies in young diabetics have reported an increased end-systolic dimension (Rubler et al, 1978; Lababidi and Goldstein, 1983), which suggested that systolic function of the left ventricle was impaired in these otherwise healthy patients. The differences in both studies were small compared to the controls, and in neither study was allowance made for possible differences in body mass. In contrast, most other studies have reported that systolic function is normal in adult diabetics when they are considered as a group (Zoneraich et al, 1977; Shapiro et al, 1981a; Shapiro, 1984). In contrast, abnormal diastolic function of the left ventricle has been emphasised by some authors (Sanderson et al, 1978; Shapiro, 1981a, 1982, 1984). Opening of the mitral valve was frequently delayed and the rapid phase of early diastolic filling was often prolonged. In some patients this was associated with a reduced rate of thinning of the left ventricular posterior wall, further supporting the concept of slow chamber filling. Although it is difficult to be certain that these changes were independent of coronary artery disease, electrocardiographic evidence of exercise-induced ischaemia was infrequently observed in these patients. Amongst 625 adult diabetics examined by Shapiro (1984), half had clinical evidence of ischaemic heart disease or hypertension; amongst those free of clinical evidence of cardiovascular disease, prolonged isovolumic relaxation with or without reduced rate of left ventricular cavity dimension increase was present in approximately one-quarter. These abnormalities were uncommon amongst diabetics free of microvascular lesions and became increasingly frequent with more severe grades of retinopathy (Sanderson, 1978; Shapiro 1982, 1984). Although it is clear that ischaemic heart disease and hypertension are commonly responsible for left ventricular dysfunction, these studies suggest that diabetic heart muscle disease may be present in an important minority of diabetics, particularly those with microvascular complications.

Haemodynamic response to exercise

Young diabetics tend to have an exaggerated pressor response to exercise. Studies in patients with juvenile onset (Type 1) diabetes revealed that although resting blood pressure (BP) was only slightly increased, the systolic pressor response during bicycle exercise was increased (Karlefors 1966): at an external workload of 900 kpm (=150 Watts), systolic blood pressure was approximately 40 mmHg higher in those with diabetes of 15 or more years duration compared to normal controls (Figure 2.2). When restudied after 8–10 years, the increased systolic blood pressure, both at rest and during exercise, was more clearly evident (Persson, 1977). Maximum achieved workload was also reduced in the diabetics, only 10 per cent being able to

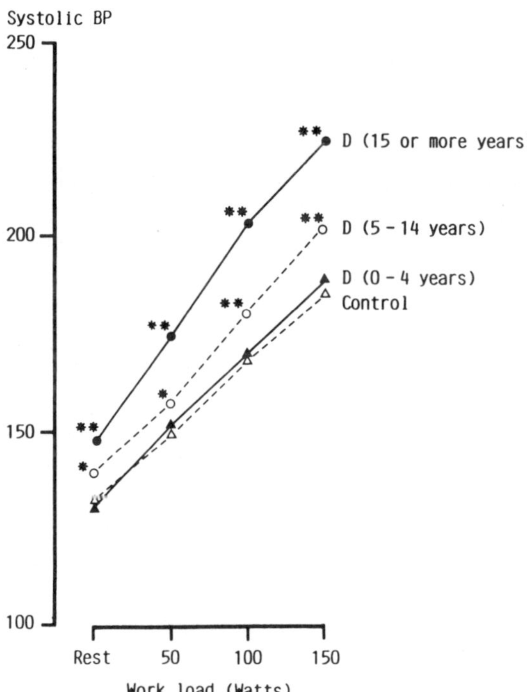

Figure 2.2 Systolic blood pressure at rest and during bicycle exercise at workloads of 50, 100 and 150 Watts in control patients and patients with diabetes of 0–4, 5–14 and more than 15 years' duration. *$p < 0.05$, **$p < 0.01$, comparing diabetics with the control group. Data derived from Karlefors (1966).

exercise at a workload of 200 Watts compared to 50 per cent of controls.

Invasive measurement of haemodynamic responses to exercise performed in 41 diabetics demonstrated that resting stroke volume tended to be lower than normal (Karlefors, 1966), especially in those with diabetes of longer than five years' duration. During exercise, the increase in cardiac output was significantly reduced compared to controls; this was due to both a smaller increment in stroke volume and a greater increase in systemic vascular resistance during exercise.

Recently, non-invasive studies using technetium ventriculography have confirmed that exercise responses are impaired in diabetes (Vered et al, 1984). After labelling of the bloodpool with technetium pertechnetate, ventricular volumes at end-systole and end-diastole can be measured to derive ejection fraction. In normal subjects, ejection fraction increases by at least 4 per cent during exercise. Amongst 30 young diabetics (mean age 30 years), half of whom were insulin-dependent, a subnormal increase in ejection fraction was observed in 44 per cent; in 17 per cent ejection fraction actually decreased during exercise. Only four patients had diabetic retinopathy, and in three of these the exercise response was abnormal. Since hypertensive diabetics were excluded and the product of heart rate and systolic blood pressure at rest and on exercise were similar in diabetics and controls, it is unlikely that these differences were due to an abnormal pressor response during exercise.

These studies indicate that in otherwise healthy diabetics, the cardiovascular response to exercise is impaired as a result of both reduced inotropic responses and a tendency towards increased total peripheral resistance during exercise.

Cardiac catheterisation

Regan and co-workers have reported detailed findings at cardiac catheterisation in 12 diabetics who were free of significant coronary artery disease (Regan et al, 1977); most patients had evidence of retinopathy; five were treated with diet, four with insulin and three with oral hypoglycaemic agents. Eight of these subjects were previously free of clinical heart failure. Compared to controls, these subjects exhibited a smaller left ventricular volume at end-diastole, together with a significantly elevated left ventricular filling pressure and a reduced left ventricular stroke volume. Similar but more marked abnormalities were observed in four diabetics who had previously developed clinical heart failure. The normal cardiac response to increased systemic vascular resistance during angiotensin II infusion was an increase in stroke volume associated with a small increase in ventricular filling pressure. In contrast, a marked rise in filling pressure without any increase in stroke volume was observed in the diabetics. Experimental studies (Regan et al, 1974) in dogs with alloxan-induced diabetes during angiotensin II infusion and volume expansion with saline demonstrated impaired stroke volume responses closely similar to those observed in the diabetic patients. These abnormal responses were attributed to a poorly compliant myocardium.

Clinical role of diabetic heart muscle disease

These studies emphasise the importance of enhanced deposition of myocardial fibrous tissue in diabetic heart muscle disease. It is tempting to suggest a unifying hypothesis whereby myocardial fibrosis may lead to abnormalities of both systolic and diastolic myocardial performance in diabetic patients, especially those with evidence of microvascular disease in other organs. Increased myocardial fibrosis might be expected to lead directly to abnormal myocardial relaxation due to a restraining effect; the resulting elevation of diastolic filling pressures would tend to lead to impaired subendocardial blood flow independent of any structural abnormality of the coronary arterial bed. Impaired systolic function may result directly from myocardial fibrosis or may be secondary to reduced compliance, preventing stretch of myocardial fibres and interference with the normal Starling response (stretching of cardiac muscle fibres normally leads to increased contractility).

Further studies are needed to clarify the evolution of left ventricular dysfunction, especially amongst insulin-dependent diabetics with developing retinopathy. The potential importance of an interaction between elevated blood pressure, especially during exercise, and left ventricular dysfunction in diabetes requires detailed prospective evaluation. The relationship between abnormalities detected by systolic time intervals and echocardiography and those detected by exercise technetium ventriculography require further evaluation.

Does diabetic heart muscle disease commonly lead to heart failure with a dilated poorly contracting heart? Diabetes is an uncommon feature in patients with primary myocardial failure (congestive cardiomyopathy). Amongst 100 consecutive patients with congestive cardiomyopathy, the prevalence of diabetes was 5 per cent, similar to that expected in this population (Hamby, 1970). Although a subsequent report, also by Hamby (Hamby et al, 1974), suggested a greater prevalence of diabetes amongst such patients, in half the diabetics glucose intolerance was mild and of short duration suggesting that it was a consequence rather than a cause of heart failure. In Shapiro's study of 625 diabetics, left ventricular failure or dilatation were observed in only 18 patients, most of whom had pre-existing hypertension or myocardial infarction (Shapiro, 1984). Thus far, there is good evidence for myocardial disease in diabetics, especially in those with retinopathy and probably closely associated with microangiopathy. Numerically, hypertension and ischaemic heart disease are likely to be much more important causes of death or myocardial failure in the diabetic than heart muscle disease alone. However, disordered myocardial function may contribute importantly to the high mortality from myocardial failure which occurs amongst diabetics with acute myocardial infarction.

Treatment of Heart Failure in Diabetes

In diabetics with clinical evidence of heart failure, treatment with loop diuretics (e.g., furosemide, bumetanide) is preferable to thiazide diuretics in view of the diabetogenic effects of the latter. Avoidance of diuretic-induced hypokalaemia (and possibly hypomagnesaemia) is important in view of the potential for inducing rhythm disturbances associated with electrolyte abnormalities. In non-diabetics potassium-sparing diuretics (e.g., triamterene, amiloride, spironolactone) are commonly used in conjunction with loop diuretics in order to prevent hypokalaemia. However, these drugs should be used with caution in diabetics since triamterene and amiloride have been reported to increase fasting blood glucose in poorly controlled diabetics and to cause a paradoxical increase in serum potassium after intravenous glucose (a similar effect occurred after oral glucose in one patient treated with triamterene) (McNay and Oran, 1970; Walker et al, 1972). In normal subjects, both insulin and aldosterone play important roles in defence against hyperkalaemia (Cox et al, 1978); co-existing deficiencies of aldosterone and insulin are not uncommon in diabetics and may compromise these defences (Christlieb et al, 1976; De Chatel et al, 1977). For example, in diabetics with suppressed plasma renin activity and aldosterone, oral glucose resulted in paradoxical increases in serum potassium (Perez et al, 1977). Therapeutic suppression of the renin–aldosterone system by drugs such as spironolactone or converting enzyme inhibitors, for example, captopril, may increase the risks of hyperkalaemia in diabetics; for these reasons, careful monitoring of serum potassium is mandatory when potassium-sparing diuretics are used in diabetic patients.

Patients with atrial fibrillation and heart failure often respond well to digoxin. When atrial fibrillation remains poorly controlled at rest or on exercise despite therapeutic plasma digoxin concentrations, cautious addition of small doses of verapamil may improve exercise tolerance (Lang et al, 1983); however, plasma digoxin levels often increase with verapamil (Klein et al, 1982) and there is a potential risk of provoking bradycardia or worsening of heart failure. Combined use of digoxin with quinidine or disopyramide may be considered in this context; again, negative inotropic effects with both drugs and increases of digoxin levels with quinidine are possible adverse effects (Bussey, 1984). In patients in sinus rhythm, digoxin may have a useful positive inotropic effect, especially in patients with marked cardiomegaly and a third heart sound (Lee et al, 1982).

Vasodilator drugs (e.g., hydralazine, prazosin, captopril, isosorbide dinitrate) have assumed an important role in the management of heart failure patients poorly responsive to diuretics or digoxin. These drugs may be dramatically effective in mitral incompetence. However, there is a risk of provoking hypotension, reducing cardiac output and exacerbating renal failure, particularly in patients with low cardiac filling pressures, often due to diuretic-induced hypovolaemia; for these reasons, these drugs should be used cautiously in heart-failure patients after careful clinical evaluation by a physician with expertise in cardiovascular disease.

Tolerance and activation of compensatory mechanisms (particularly activation of the renin–angiotensin system) may lead to attenuation of the beneficial haemodynamic effects during long-term treatment with some drugs, particularly prazosin and isosorbide dinitrate. Converting enzyme inhibitors, such as captopril, appear to have a sustained haemodynamic effect (Bayliss et al, 1985) which in the future may lead to these drugs having a well-established therapeutic role. However, converting enzyme inhibitors have not been specifically evaluated in diabetics with heart failure and, in view of the potential for hyperkalaemia, they should be used with caution at present.

Diabetic Autonomic Neuropathy and the Cardiovascular System

Troublesome symptoms such as postural dizziness, diarrhoea, hypoglycaemic unawareness, abnormal sweating, disturbed bladder function, impotence and gastric fullness are well recognised to occur in diabetics with autonomic neuropathy. During the last decade, reliable non-invasive tests assessing autonomic control of the cardiovascular system have been extensively evaluated. Among patients with symptomatic autonomic dysfunction, these tests of cardiovascular function are nearly always abnormal, confirming that the symptoms reflect widespread autonomic neuropathy; however, in patients with impotence, abnormal tests are uncommon, suggesting that this symptom correlates poorly with autonomic dysfunction (Ewing et al, 1980; Clarke & Ewing, 1982).

Table 2.3 summarises the tests which have been extensively evaluated and found to be of greatest clinical application. The heart-rate response to deep breathing tests only vagally mediated heart-rate responses; since vagal tone declines with age, it is important to make allowance for age in determining the normal range (Smith, 1982; Wieling et al, 1982; Masaoka et al, 1985). Heart-rate responses to standing and the Valsalva manoeuvre require more coopera-

tion from the patient and reflect complex integrated responses involving vagally mediated heart-rate changes as well as sympathetically mediated heart-rate and peripheral vasoconstrictor responses (Korner et al, 1976; Borst et al, 1982). Similarly, blood-pressure responses to handgrip exercise predominantly assess sympathetic vasoconstrictor responses as well as heart-rate-mediated changes in cardiac output (Ewing et al, 1974; Nazar et al, 1975).

Studies of diabetics without symptoms of autonomic neuropathy have demonstrated that these tests are frequently abnormal, particularly in patients with either evidence of microvascular complications (Mackay et al, 1980; Dryberg et al, 1981) (retinopathy, nephropathy) or clinical evidence of somatic neuropathy (Masaoka et al, 1985). Heart-rate responses to deep breathing are most frequently abnormal (Dryberg et al, 1981) (30–40 per cent), followed by abnormal responses to standing and Valsalva's manoeuvre (about 20 per cent); abnormal blood-pressure responses to postural change and handgrip are infrequent. More recently (Ewing et al, 1984), computer analysis of 24-hour electrocardiograph recordings have shown that sudden transient

Table 2.3 Tests of autonomic function and normal ranges

Test	*Assess*	*Results*		
		Normal	*Borderline*	*Abnormal*
Heart-rate variation				
Deep breathing (6/min)	Average heart rate range over 5 beats (beats/min) (Ewing et al, 1980)	>15	11–14	<10
Valsalva manoeuvre (40 mmHg × 15 sec)	Valsalva ratio (ratio of maximum heart rate during manoeuvre to minimum heart rate after release) (Korner et al, 1976)	>1.21	1.11–1.2	<1.10
Lying to standing	30 : 15 ratio (ratio of 30th to 15th RR′ interval from onset of standing) (Ewing et al, 1980)	>1.04	1.01–1.03	<1.00
Blood-pressure change				
Lying to standing	Systolic fall (mmHg) (Ewing et al, 1980; Borst et al, 1982)	<10	11–29	≥30
Sustained handgrip (30% maximum × 4–5 min)	Diastolic rise (mmHg) (Ewing et al, 1974)	>16	11–15	≤10

changes in pulse interval ($>$50 msec) occur commonly in normal subjects and are thought to reflect vagal control of heart rate; among diabetics with normal heart-rate responses to autonomic tests, patients were identified who had a reduced number of pulse interval transitions suggesting that parasympathetic dysfunction may be even more common than previously suspected. The high frequency of abnormal tests of vagal function and the low prevalence of abnormal tests of sympathetic function (nearly always accompanied by abnormal vagal tests) have led some workers to suggest that vagal neuropathy develops early, while sympathetic neuropathy is a late complication. On the other hand, more recent evidence suggests the possibility of early sympathetic impairment among patients with abnormal heart-rate responses to breathing without impaired blood-pressure responses to posture (Hilsted et al, 1979, 1980). These subjects were found to have a reduced physical working capacity; heart-rate and blood-pressure responses and plasma catecholamine, cortisol and growth-hormone responses were found to be impaired when expressed in terms of the subject's maximum oxygen uptake. These observations suggest that the cardiovascular and endocrine reserve of such patients may be substantially limited during stress.

Clinical implications

Follow-up of patients with symptomatic autonomic neuropathy and abnormal function tests indicated a very poor prognosis with a calculated five-year mortality rate of 56 per cent (Ewing et al, 1980). Approximately half of the deaths were related to diabetic nephropathy; however, nine of the 26 deaths in these patients were cardiovascular (sudden deaths five, stroke three, myocardial infarction one), and it has been speculated that sudden death may be a specific complication of diabetic autonomic neuropathy. Page and Watkins (1978) reported that cardiorespiratory arrest occurred commonly amongst diabetics with autonomic neuropathy, particularly after anaesthesia, and recommended careful monitoring of such patients after surgery or during illnesses which might interfere with respiratory drive. An increased frequency of sleep apnoea has been reported in two studies (Guilleminault et al, 1981; Rees et al, 1981) of patients with autonomic neuropathy which included diabetics; however, a further study was unable to confirm these observations (Catterall et al, 1984).

Disturbances in cardiac innervation may predispose to ventricular arrhythmias. In animal studies intact vagal innervation can be shown to protect against ventricular arrhythmias occurring during sympathetic stimulation and ischaemia. Following recovery from myocardial infarction in dogs, exercise and ischaemia provoked ventricular fibrillation more commonly in dogs with poor baroreflex function (largely vagally mediated) than in those with preserved responses (Billman et al, 1982). Studies of patients with the long QT syndrome who are susceptible to ventricular arrhythmias indicate the decisive importance of the balance between the right and the left cardiac sympathetic nerves in man (Schwartz & Stone, 1982). It is possible that the combination of vagal denervation and patchy cardiac sympathetic denervation might provide an excellent setting for the development of major ventricular arrhythmias in diabetics with cardiac autonomic denervation.

Study of the diabetic may provide further insight into the role of the autonomic nervous system in cardiovascular control and may lead to important therapeutic strategies.

References

Abenavoli, T., Rubler, S., Fisher, V.J. et al (1981). Exercise testing with myocardial scintigraphy in asymptomatic diabetic males. *Circulation* **63**, 54–64.

Abrams, J. (1984). The brief saga of transdermal nitroglycerin discs: paradise lost? *Am. J. Cardiol.* **54**, 220–224.

Ahmed, S.S., Jaferi, G.A., Narang, R.M. et al (1975). Preclinical abnormality of left ventricular function in diabetes mellitus. *Am. Heart J.* **89**, 153–158.

Alpert, M.A. and Flaker G.C. (1984). Chronic fascicular blocks. Recognition, natural history and therapeutic considerations. *Arch. Intern. Med.* **144**, 799–802.

Anon (1982). Long term and short term beta-blockade after myocardial infarction. *Lancet* **i**, 1159–1161.

Baber, N.S., Julian, D.G., Lewis, J.A. et al (1984). ß-Blockers after myocardial infarction: have trials changed practice? *Br. Med. J.* **289**, 1431–1432.

Bayliss, J., Norell, M.S., Canepa-Anson, R. et al (1985). Clinical importance of the renin-angiotensin system in chronic heart failure: double-blind comparison of captopril and prazosin. *Br. Med. J.* **290**, 1861–1865.

Bhatnagar, S.K., Amin, M.M.A. & Al.Yusuf, A.R. (1984). Diabetogenic effects of nifedipine. *Br. Med. J.* **289**, 19.

Billman, G.E., Schwartz, P.J. and Stone, H.L. (1982). Baroreceptor reflex control of heart rate: a predictor of sudden cardiac death. *Circulation* **66**, 874–880.

Bisset, G.S., Schwartz, D.C., Meyer, R.A. (1980). Clinical spectrum and longterm follow-up of isolated mitral valve prolapse in 119 children. *Circulation* **62**, 423–429.

Blandford, R.L. and Burden, A.C. (1984). Abnormalities of cardiac conduction in diabetics. *Br. Med.J.* **289**, 1659.

Blumenthal, H.T., Alex, M. and Goldenberg, S. (1960). A study of lesions of the intramural coronary artery branches in diabetes mellitus. *Arch. Pathol.* **70**, 27–41.

Borst, C., Wieling, W., van Brederobe, J.F.M. et al (1982). Mechanisms of initial heart rate response to postural change. *Am. J. Physiol* **242**, H676–681.

Bussey, H.I. (1984). Update on the influence of quinidine and other agents on digitalis glycosides. *Am. Heart J.* **107**, 143–146.

CASS Principal Investigators and their Associates (1983). Coronary artery surgery study (CASS): a randomized trial of coronary artery by-pass surgery. Survival data. *Circulation* **68**, 939–950.

Catterall, J.R., Calverley, P.M.A., Ewing, D.J. et al (1984). Breathing, sleep and diabetic autonomic neuropathy. *Diabetes* **33**, 1025–1027.

Chamberlain, D.A. (1983). Beta-adrenoceptor blockers after acute myocardial infarction—where are we now? *Br. Heart J.* **49**, 105–110.

Charles, S., Ketelslegers, J-M., Buysschaert, M. et al (1981). Hyperglycaemic effect of nifedipine. *Br. Med. J.* **283**, 19–20.

Christlieb, A.R., Kaldany, A. and D'Elia, J.A. (1976). Plasma renin activity and hypertension in diabetes mellitus. *Diabetes* **25**, 969–974.

Chychota, N.N., Gau, G.T., Pluth, J.R. et al (1973). Myocardial revascularization. Comparison of operability and surgical results in diabetic and non-diabetic patients. *J. Thorac. Cardiovasc. Surg.* **65**, 856–862.

Clark, R.S., English, M., McNeill, G.P. et al (1985). Effect of intravenous infusion of insulin in diabetics with acute myocardial infarction. *Br. Med. J.* **291**, 303–305.

Clarke, B.F. and Ewing, D.J. (1982). Cardiovascular reflex tests. *NY State J. Med.* **82**, 903–908.

Cox, M., Sterns, R.H. and Singer, I. (1978). The defense against hyperkalaemia: the roles of insulin and aldosterone. *N. Engl. J. Med.* **299**, 525–531.

Crall, F.R. and Roberts, W.C. (1978). The extramural and intramural coronary arteries in juvenile diabetes mellitus. *Am. J. Med.* **64**, 221–230.

Czyzk, A., Krolewski, A.S., Szablowska, S. et al (1980). Clinical course of myocardial infarction among diabetic patients. *Diabetes Care* **3**, 526–529.

Deacon, S.P. and Barnett, D. (1976). Comparison of atenolol and propranolol during insulin-induced hypoglycaemia. *Br. Med. J.* **2**, 272–273.

Deacon, S.P., Karunanayake, A. and Barnett, D. (1977). Acebutolol, atenolol and propranolol and metabolic responses to acute hypoglycaemia in diabetics. *Br. Med. J.* **2**, 1255–1257.

De Chatel, R., Weidmann, P., Flammer, F. et al (1977). Sodium, renin, aldosterone, catecholamines and blood pressure in diabetes mellitus. *Kidney Int.* **12**, 412–421.

Donnelly, T. and Harrower, A.D.B. (1980). Effect of nifedipine on glucose tolerance and insulin secretion in diabetic and non-diabetic patients. *Curr. Med. Res. Opin.* **6**, 690–693.

Dornhorst, A., Powell, S.H. and Pensky, J. (1985). Aggravation by propranolol of hyperglycaemic effect of hydrochlorothiazide in type II diabetics without alteration of insulin secretion. *Lancet* **i**, 123–126.

Dortimer, A.C., Shenoy, P.N., Shiroff, R.A. et al (1978). Diffuse coronary artery disease in diabetic patients. Fact or fiction? *Circulation* **57**, 133–136.

Dryberg, T., Benn, J., Christiansen, J.S. et al (1981). Prevalence of diabetic autonomic neuropathy measured by simple bedside tests. *Diabetologia* **20**, 190–194.

Engleman, R.M., Bhat, J.G., Glassman, E. et al (1976). The influence of diabetes and hypertension on the results of coronary revascularization. *Am. J. Med. Sci.* **271**, 4–12.

European Coronary Surgery Study Group (1982). Longterm results of prospective randomised study of coronary artery bypass surgery in stable angina pectoris. *Lancet* **ii**, 1173–1180.

Ewing, D.J., Borsey, D.Q., Travis, P. et al (1983). Abnormalities of ambulatory 24-hour heart rate in diabetes mellitus. *Diabetes* **32**, 101–105.

Ewing, D.J., Campbell, I.W. and Clarke, B.F. (1980). The natural history of diabetic autonomic neuropathy. *Q.J. Med.* **49**, 95–108.

Ewing, D.J., Irving, J.B., Kerr, F. et al (1974). Cardiovascular responses to sustained handgrip in normal subjects and in patients with diabetes mellitus: a test of autonomic function. *Clin. Sci.* **46**, 295–306.

Ewing, D.J., Neilson, J.M.M. and Travis, P. (1984). New method for assessing cardiac parasympathetic activity using 24 hour electrocardiograms. *Br. Heart J.* **52**, 396–402.

Factor, S.M., Minase, T. and Sonnenblick, E.H. (1980 a). Clinical and morphological features of human hypertensive diabetic cardiomyopathy. *Am. Heart J.* **99**, 446–458.

Factor, S.M., Okun, E.M. and Minase, T. (1980b). Capillary microaneurysms in the human diabetic heart. *N. Engl. J. Med.* **302**, 384–388.

Fairfax, A.J. and Leatham, A. (1975). Idiopathic heart block: association with vitiligo, thyroid disease, pernicious anaemia and diabetes mellitus. *Br. Med. J.* **4** 322–324.

Fein, F.S., Capasso, J.M., Aronson, R.S. et al (1984). Combined renovascular hypertension and diabetes in rats: a new preparation of congestive cardiomyopathy. *Circulation* **70**, 318–330.

Fischer, V.W., Barner, H.B. and Leskiw, M.L. (1979). Capillary basal laminar thickness in diabetic human myocardium. *Diabetes* **28**, 713–719.

Friedman, N.E., Levitsky, L.L., Edidin, D.V. et al (1982). Echocardiographic evidence for impaired myocardial performance in children with Type I diabetes mellitus. *Am. J. Med.* **73**, 846–850.

Fuller, J.H., Shipley, M.J., Rose, G. et al (1980). Coronary heart disease risk and impaired glucose tolerance. The Whitehall Study. *Lancet* **ii**, 1373–1376.

Garcia, M.J., McNamara, P.M., Gordon, T. et al (1974). Morbidity and mortality in diabetics in the Framingham Population. Sixteen year follow-up study. *Diabetes* **23**, 105–111.

Giugliano, D., Gentile, S., Verza, M. et al (1981). Modulation by verapamil of insulin and glucagon secretion in man. *Acta Diabetol. Lat.* **18**, 163–171.

Giugliano, D., Torella, R., Cacciapuoti, F. et al (1980). Impairment of insulin secretion in man by nifedipine. *Eur. J. Clin. Pharmacol.* **18**, 395–398.

Goodwin, J.F. (1972). Congestive and hypertrophic cardiomyopathies; a decade of study. *Br. Heart J.* **34**, 545–552.

Greenwood, R.H. (1982). Hypoglycaemic effect of nifedipine. *Br. Med. J.* **284**, 50.

Guilleminault, C., Briskin, J.G., Greenfield, M.S. et al (1981). The impact of autonomic nervous system dysfunction on breathing during sleep. *Sleep* **4**, 263–278.

Gundersen, T. and Kjekshus, J. (1983). Timolol treatment after myocardial infarction in diabetic patients. *Diabetics Care* **6**, 285–290.

Gwilt, D.J., Petri, M., Lamb, P. et al (1984a). Effect of intravenous insulin infusion on mortality among diabetic patients after myocardial infarction. *Br. Heart J.* **51**, 626–630.

Gwilt, D.J., Petri, M., Lewis, P.W. et al (1984b). Infarct size and mortality in diabetic patients. *Br. Heart J.* **51**, 680P.

Hamby, R.I. (1970). Primary myocardial disease: a prospective clinical and hemodynamic evaluation of 100 patients. *Medicine* **49**, 55–78.

Hamby, R.I., Zoneraich, S. and Sherman, L. (1974). Diabetic cardiomyopathy. *JAMA* **229**, 1749–1754.

Harrower, A.D.B. and Clarke, B.F. (1976). Experience of coronary care in diabetes. *Br. Med. J.* **1**, 126–128.

Hasslacher, C. and Wahl, P. (1977). Diabetes prevalence in patients with bradycardiac arrhythmias. *Acta Diabetol. Lat.* **14**, 229–234.

Hilsted, J., Galbo, H. and Christensen, N-J. (1979). Impaired cardiovascular responses to graded exercise in diabetic autonomic neuropathy. *Diabetes* **28**, 313–319.

Hilsted, J., Galbo, H. and Christensen, N-J. (1980). Impaired responses of catecholamines, growth hormone and cortisol to graded exercise in diabetic autonomic neuropathy. *Diabetes* **29**, 257–262.

Hjalmarson, A., Elmfeldt, D., Herlitz, J. et al (1981). Effect on mortality of metoprolol in acute myocardial infarction. *Lancet* **ii**, 823–826.

Hosenpud, I.D., Montanaro, A., Hart, M.V. et al (1984). Myocardial perfusion abnormalities in asymptomatic patients with systemic lupus erythematosus. *Am. J. Med.* **77**, 286–292.

Jaffe, B.I., Lamprey, J.M., Shires, R. et al (1983). Lack of hormonal effects of a single dose of nifedipine in healthy young men. *J. Cardiovasc. Pharmacol.* **5**, 700–702.

Jaffe, A.S., Spadaro, J.J., Schechtman, K. et al (1984). Increased congestive heart failure after myocardial infarction of modest extent in patients with diabetes mellitus. *Am. Heart. J.* **108**, 31–37.

Johnson, W.D., Pedraza, P.M. and Kayser, K.L. (1982). Coronary artery surgery in diabetics: 261 consecutive patients followed 4 to 7 years. *Am. Heart J.* **104**, 823–827.

Kannel, W.B. and McGee, D.L. (1979). Diabetes and cardiovascular disease. The Framingham Study. *JAMA* **241**, 2035–2038.

Karlefors, T. (1966). Circulatory studies during exercise with particular reference to diabetics. *Acta. Med. Scand.* **180**, Suppl. 449.

Klein, H.O., Lang, R., Weiss, E. et al (1982). The influence of verapamil on serum drug concentration. *Circulation* **65**, 998–1003.

Korner, P.I., Tonkin, A.M. and Uther, J.B. (1976). Reflex and mechanical circulatory effects of graded

Valsalva manoeuvres in normal man. *J. Appl. Physiol.* **40**, 434–440.

Lababidi, Z.A. and Goldstein, D.E. (1983). High prevalence of echocardiographic abnormalities in diabetic youths. *Diabetes care* **6**, 18–22.

Laffel, G.L. and Braunwald, E. (1984). Thrombolytic therapy. A new strategy for the treatment of acute myocardial infarction. *N. Engl. J. Med.* **311**, 710–717, 770–776.

Lager, I., Blohme, G. and Smith, V. (1979). Effect of cardioselective and non-selective ß-blockade on the hypoglycaemic response in insulin-dependent diabetics. *Lancet* **i**, 458–462.

Lang, R., Klein H.O., Weiss, E. et al (1983). Superiority of oral verapamil to digoxin in treatment of chronic atrial fibrillation. *Chest* **83**, 491–499.

Ledet, T. (1976). Diabetic cardiopathy: quantitative histological studies of the heart from young juvenile diabetics. *Acta Pathol. Microbiol.* **84**, Section A, 421–428.

Ledet, T. (1968). Histological and histochemical changes in the coronary arteries of old diabetic patients. *Diabetologia* **4**, 268–272.

Lee, D.C., Johnson, R.A. and Bingham, J.B. (1982). Heart failure in outpatients. A randomised trial of digoxin versus placebo. *N. Engl. J. Med.* **306**, 699–705.

Lloyd-Mostyn, R.H. and Oram, S. (1975). Modification by propranolol of cardiovascular effects of insulin-induced hypoglycaemia. *Lancet* **i**, 1213–1215.

Mackay, J.D., Page, M.Mc.B., Cambridge, J. et al (1980). Diabetic autonomic neuropathy. *Diabetologia* **18**, 471–478.

McNeer, J.F., Margolis, J.R., Lee, K.L. et al (1978). The role of the exercise test in the evaluation of patients with ischaemic heart disease. *Circulation* **57**, 64–70.

McNay, J.L. and Oran, E. (1970). Possible predisposition of diabetic patients to hyperkalaemia following administration of potassium retaining diuretic, Amiloride (MK 870). *Metabolism* **19**, 58–70.

Margolis, J.L. Krieger, J. and Glemser, E. (1984). Coronary angioplasty: increased restenosis rate in insulin dependent diabetics. *Circulation* **70**, Suppl. 2, 175.

Masaoka, S., Lev-Ran, A., Hill, L.R. et al (1985). Heart rate variability in diabetes: relationship to age and duration of the disease. *Diabetes Care* **8**, 64–68.

MIAMI Trial Research Group (1985). Metoprolol in acute myocardial infarction (MIAMI). A randomised placebo-controlled international trial. *Eur. Heart J.* **6**, 199–226.

Nazar, K., Taton, J., Chwalbinska-Moneta, J. et al (1975). Adrenergic responses to sustained handgrip in patients with juvenile onset type diabetes mellitus. *Clin. Sci. Mol. Med.* **49**, 39–44.

Nicod, P., Lewis, S.E., Corbett, J.C. et al (1982). Increased incidence and clinical correlation of persistently abnormal technetium pyrophosphate myocardial scintigrams following acute myocardial infarction in patients with diabetes mellitus. *Am. Heart J.* **103**, 822–829.

Norwegian Multicenter Study Group (1981). Timolol-induced reduction in mortality and reinfarction in patients surviving acute myocardial infarction. *N. Engl. J. Med.* **304**, 801–807.

Page, M.Mc.B. and Watkins, P.J. (1978). Cardio-respiratory arrest and diabetic autonomic neuropathy. *Lancet* **i**, 14–16.

Partamian, J.O. and Bradley, R.F. (1965). Acute myocardial infarction in 258 cases of diabetes. *N. Engl. J. Med.* **273**, 455–461.

Perez, G.O., Lespier, L., Knowles, R. et al (1977). Potassium homeostasis in chronic diabetes mellitus. *Arch. Intern. Med.* **137**, 1018–1022.

Persson, G. (1977). Exercise test in male diabetics. *Acta Med. Scand.* Suppl. 605, 7–23.

Posner, J., Ilya, R., Wanderman, K. et al (1983). Systolic time intervals in diabetes. *Diabetologia* **24**, 249–252.

Rees, P.J., Prior, J.G., Cochrane, G.M. et al (1981). Sleep apnoea in diabetic patients with autonomic neuropathy. *J. R. Soc. Med.* **74**, 192–195.

Regan, T.J., Ettinger, P.O., Khan, M.I. et al (1974). Altered myocardial function and metabolism in chronic diabetes mellitus without ischaemia in dogs. *Circ. Res.* **35**, 222–237.

Regan, T.J., Lyons, M.M., Ahmed, S.S. et al (1977). Evidence for cardiomyopathy in familial diabetes mellitus. *J. Clin. Invest.* **60**, 885–899.

Riley, C.G., Oberman, A. and Sheffield, L.T. (1972). Electrocardiographic effects of glucose ingestion. *Arch. Intern. Med.* **130**, 703–707.

Rojdmark, S. and Andersson, D.E.H. (1984). Influence of verapamil on glucose tolerance. *Acta Med. Scand.* **215**, Suppl. 681, 37–42.

Rubler, S., Dlugash, J., Yuceoglu, Y.E. et al (1972). New type of cardiomyopathy associated with diabetic glomerulosclerosis. *Am. J. Cardiol.* **30**, 595–602.

Rubler, S., Sajadi, M.R.M., Araoye, M.A. et al (1978). Non-invasive estimation of myocardial performance in patients with diabetes. Effect of alcohol administration. *Diabetes* **27**, 127–134.

Sanderson, J.E., Brown, D.J., Rivellese, A. et al (1978). Diabetic cardiomyopathy? An echocardiographic study of young diabetics. *Br. Med. J.* **2**, 404–407.

Schwartz, P.J. and Stone, H.L. (1982). The role of the autonomic nervous system in sudden coronary death. *Ann. NY Acad. Sci.* **382**, 162–180.

Seneviratne, B.I.B. (1977). Diabetic cardiomyopathy: the preclinical phase. *Br. Med. J.* **1**, 1444–1446.

Shapiro, L.M. (1982). Echocardiographic features of impaired ventricular function in diabetes mellitus. *Br. Heart J.* **47**, 439–444.

Shapiro, L.M. (1984). A prospective study of heart disease in diabetes mellitus. *Q. J. Med.* **209**, 55–68.

Shapiro, L.M., Howat, A.P. and Calter, M.M. (1981a). Left ventricular function in diabetes mellitus. I: Methodology, prevalence and spectrum of abnormalities. *Br. Heart J.* **45**, 122–128.

Shapiro, L.M., Leatherdale, B.A., Mackinnon, J. et al (1981b). Left ventricular function in diabetes mellitus. II: Relationship between clinical features and left ventricular function. *Br. Heart. J.* **45**, 129–132.

Smith, J.W., Marcus, F.I. & Sorokman, R. (1984). Prognosis of patients with diabetes mellitus after acute myocardial infarction. *Am. J. Cardiol.* **54**, 718–721.

Smith, S.A. (1982). Reduced sinus arrhythmia in diabetic autonomic neuropathy: diagnostic value of an age-related normal range. *Br. Med. J.* **2**, 1599–1601.

Soler, N.G., Bennett, M.A., Lamb, P. et al (1974). Coronary care for myocardial infarction in diabetics. *Lancet* **i**, 475–477.

Soler, N.G., Bennett, M.A., Pentecost, B.L. et al (1975). Myocardial infarction in diabetics. *Q. J. Med.* **44**, 125–132.

Stewart, W.J., McSweeney, S.M., Kellett, M.A. et al (1984). Increased risk of severe protamine reactions in NPH insulin-dependent diabetics undergoing cardiac catheterisation. *Circulation* **70**, 788–792.

Sykes, C.A., Wright, A.D., Malins, J.M. et al (1977). Changes in systolic time intervals during treatment of diabetes mellitus. *Br. Heart J.* **39**, 255–259.

Taggart, P., Carruthers, M., Joseph, S. et al (1979). Electrocardiographic changes resembling myocardial ischaemia in asymptomatic men with normal coronary arteriograms. *Br. Heart J.* **41**, 214–225.

Tansey, M.J.B., Opie, L.H. & Kennelly, B.M. (1977). High mortality in obese women diabetics with acute myocardial infarction. *Br. Med. J.* **1**, 1624–1626.

Uusitupa, M., Siitonen, O., Aro, A. et al (1983). Effect of correction of hyperglycaemia on left ventricular function in non-insulin-dependent (type 2) diabetics. *Acta Med. Scand.* **213**, 363–268.

Vered, Z., Battler, A., Segal, P. et al (1984). Exercise-induced left ventricular dysfunction in young men with asymptomatic diabetes mellitus (diabetic cardiomyopathy). *Am. J. Cardiol.* **54**, 633–637.

Verska, J.J. and Walker, W.J. (1975). Aortocoronary bypass in the diabetic patient. *Am. J. Cardiol.* **35**, 774–777.

Walker, B.R., Capuzzi, D.M. Alexander, F. et al (1972). Hyperkalaemia after triamterene in diabetic patients. *Clin. Pharmacol. Ther.* **13**, 643–651.

Walker, W.S., Reid, K.G., Hider, C.F. et al (1984). Successful cardiopulmonary bypass in diabetics with anaphylactoid reactions to protamine. *Br. Heart J.* **52**, 112–114.

Waller, B.F., Palumbo, P.J., Lie, J.T. et al (1980). Status of the coronary arteries in diabetes mellitus with onset after age 30 years. *Am. J. Med.* **69**, 498–506.

Wieling, W., van Brederode, J.F.M., de Rijk, L.G. et al (1982). Reflex control of heart rate in normal subjects in relation to age: a data base for cardiac vagal neuropathy. *Diabetologia* **22**, 163–166.

Willman, V.L. (1985). Percutaneous transluminal coronary angioplasty: a 1985 perspective. *Circulation* **71**, 189–192.

Wright, A.D., Barber, S.G., Kendall, M.J. et al (1979). ß-Adrenoceptor blocking drugs and blood sugar control in diabetes mellitus. *Br. Med. J.* **1**, 159–161.

Yusuf, S., Peto, R., Lewis, J. et al (1985). Beta-blockade during and after myocardial infarction: an overview of the randomised trials. *Prog. Cardiovasc. Dis.* **17**, 335–371.

Zezulka, A.V., Gill, J.S. & Beevers, D.G. (1984). Diabetogenic effects of nifedipine. *Br. Med. J.* **289**, 437–438.

Zoneraich, S., Silverman, G. and Zoneraich, O. (1980). Primary myocardial disease, diabetes mellitus and small vessel disease. *Am. Heart J.* **100**, 754–755.

Zoneraich, S., Zoneraich, O and Rhee, J.J. (1977). Left ventricular performance in diabetic patients without clinical heart disease. Evaluation by systolic time intervals and echocardiography. *Chest* **72**, 748–751.

Chapter Three

Hypertension and Diabetes Mellitus

P.J. Pacy

Dr Paul Pacy qualified from St George's Hospital, London, in 1976. He moved to Birmingham for his early clinical experience and to research on aspects of hypertension in diabetes which formed his MD thesis. He is now pursuing his clinical and research interests in diabetes and metabolism at the Clinical Research Centre, Harrow.

Introduction

Epidemiological studies, mainly in the non-diabetic, have demonstrated that hypertension is one of several major risk factors for atherosclerosis (Keys, 1975; Miller et al, 1981).

Since the widespread use of insulin therapy during the 1920s, macrovascular disease has become the major cause of morbidity and mortality in the diabetic subject in both the UK and USA (Entmacher et al, 1964; Marble, 1976; Tunbridge, 1981). Any attempt to improve the prognosis of diabetics must address this central observation. This chapter will attempt to delineate the relationship between hypertension and diabetes with specific reference to prevalence, effect on prognosis, pathophysiological mechanisms and treatment.

Prevalence of Hypertension in Diabetes

It is often claimed that hypertension is prevalent in diabetic subjects (Christlieb, 1982), although the evidence for such a statement is conflicting and by no means universally accepted.

An association between hypertension and diabetes has been suspected for over 70 years. As early as 1907 it was reported that there was a frequent association between hyperglycaemia, hypertension, atherosclerosis and obesity (Elliott, 1907). Several years later it was observed that 39 per cent of 500 diabetic patients had systolic blood pressure greater than 150 mm Hg (Kramer, 1928), and in the same year another study showed that hypertension was almost three times more common in diabetics than non-diabetics (Bell & Clawson, 1928). By the end of the 1920s the majority of published work suggested that hypertension was more prevalent in diabetics (Major, 1929); however, such a view was by no means unanimous. John (1932) found that hypertension was only more prevalent in diabetics who were over 40 years of age, while another study failed to confirm an excess prevalence (Sherrill, 1933). However, numerous methodological problems arising in these papers make comparison of the results extremely difficult. These problems include failure to standardise the definition of hypertension and diabetes, the use of either IV or V Korotkoff phases for diastolic blood pressure and a failure to take account of obesity or differentiate between the types of diabetes.

More recent studies have managed to overcome several of these problems. Pell & D'Alonzo reported that hypertension was more frequent in diabetics at 37 per cent prevalence compared to matched non-diabetics at 24 per cent, employed at the Dupont Electric Company (Pell & D'Alonzo, 1967). They also demonstrated that such differences in hypertension were present in the prediabetic state. In contrast, a large clinic-based survey failed to show similar findings and the authors felt that hypertension was no more common in diabetics than non-diabetics (Keen et al, 1975). Several large population-based surveys have confirmed that the blood pressure in diabetics is higher than in non-diabetics (Ostrander et al, 1965; Kannel & McGee, 1979), the difference being more marked in females. In addition, two recent American studies — one from a diabetic clinic population (Christlieb et al, 1981), the other a community-based study in elderly subjects (Barrett-Connor et al, 1981)— appeared to confirm the excess frequency of hypertension in diabetes. Importantly, in the community-based study the higher level of systolic blood pressure in diabetic subjects persisted even after correcting for obesity, although the relationship was not as strong.

Several large population surveys have shown an independent relationship between blood glucose and blood pressure with ethnic differences between whites and blacks also apparent (Dunn et al, 1970; Sive et al, 1971). The prevalence of hypertension is significantly greater in non-diabetic blacks than whites (Comstock, 1957; Hypertension Detection and Follow-up Program Co-operative Group, 1977), and similar findings have been confirmed in a recent clinic survey of diabetics at a District General Hospital (Pacy et al, 1985). Forty per cent (203/507) of diabetics under 65 years of age were hypertensive using the current World Health Organisation criteria (systolic blood pressure $\geqslant$ 160 mm Hg, diastolic blood pressure $\geqslant$ 95 mm Hg; World Health Organisation, 1979). Blacks (48.9 per cent) had a greater prevalence than whites (37.5 per cent ($P<0.05$) and Asians (35.4 per cent ($P<0.05$). Females (49.1 per cent) had a greater prevalence than males (33.0 per cent) ($P<0.001$), a trend noted for all ethnic groups. Those not receiving insulin therapy had a greater prevalence (45.6 per cent) than those on insulin (30.7 per cent) ($P<0.001$), although this relationship was not found in blacks in whom the prevalence of hypertension was similar regardless of the type of diabetic therapy. As in several previous studies, isolated systolic hypertension was the commonest finding (Epstein et al, 1965; Garcia et al, 1974, Hawthorne et al, 1974; Kannel & McGee, 1979) and isolated diastolic hypertension the least common in all ethnic groups. Multiple regression analysis showed a positive relationship between age and systolic ($P<0.00001$) and diastolic ($P<0.00001$) blood pressure and a negative relationship between duration of diabetes and diastolic blood pressure. ($P<0.004$). A control non-diabetic group was not recruited in this study so that it was not possible to determine whether the prevalence of hypertension in diabetics was greater than in non-diabetics. However, available data from non-diabetic populations in the age range surveyed in the diabetic clinic study have revealed prevalence rates in both sexes of between 20 and 25 per cent (Epstein et al, 1965; Garcia et al, 1974; Hawthorne et al, 1974; Kannel & McGee, 1979) which would suggest that in non-insulin-treated diabetics at least hyper-tension is more prevalent than in non-diabetics in all ethnic groups.

Although all these studies have been conducted in adult subjects, it appears that higher levels of systolic blood pressure are present in adolescent diabetics compared to non-diabetics both in Europe (Florey et al, 1976) and the USA (Moss, 1962).

The majority of data indicate that hypertension is prevalent in diabetics and at all ages their systolic blood pressure is probably higher than in non-diabetics. Evidence of higher levels of diastolic blood pressure at least before middle age is lacking, provided there is no evidence of renal impairment.

Prognosis of the Hypertensive Diabetic

The majority of evidence appears to support the concept that hypertension has an adverse effect on prognosis in the diabetic. A greater mortality in hypertensive compared to normotensive diabetics was reported in one study but no comparison with non-diabetic hypertensives was made (Hayward & Lucena, 1965), while a 10-year prospective study of 370 diabetics showed that hypertension was no more hazardous in diabetics than non-diabetics (Pell & D'Alonzo, 1970). In contrast, data from life insurance applicants suggested that for comparable degrees of hypertension the impact on mortality was greater in diabetics, and particularly marked in those aged less than 40 years (Goodkin, 1975).

The Framingham study (Kannel & McGee, 1979) has revealed that female diabetics have a 4-fold and males a 2-fold increased mortality compared to age- and sex-matched non-diabetics. In addition, coronary artery disease, cerebrovascular accidents and in particular intermittent claudication occurred more frequently in diabetics of both sexes. However, this study demonstrated that the increased prevalence of macrovascular complications was not accounted for by the increased frequency of cardiovascular risk factors including hypertension. Similar findings had previously been reported from the Joslin Clinic in the USA, although the specific role of hypertension was not evaluated (Kessler, 1971).

Evidence of a detrimental effect of hypertension has been derived from the Whitehall male civil servant study (Fuller et al, 1983). A non-linear relationship was observed between coronary heart and stroke mortality with the two hour postprandial blood glucose. Diabetics and those with postprandial blood glucose levels between 5.4–11.0 mmol/l had increased mortality compared to those with blood glucose <5.4 mmol/l. Age and hypertension were most strongly related to coronary heart and stroke mortality within both the diabetic and glucose-intolerant groups. Therefore it appears that hypertension has an additive deleterious effect on overall prognosis in the diabetic.

Classification of Hypertension

As in the non-diabetic the hypertension in diabetes can be divided into primary (essential) and secondary. Despite numerous secondary conditions (i.e., acromegaly, Cushing's and Conn's syndromes, phaeochromocytoma and thyrotoxicosis) in which elevated blood pressure is associated with impaired carbohydrate metabolism, these are probably no more frequent in the diabetic than the non-diabetic hypertensive. Likewise, other conditions, such as renal artery stenosis secondary to atherosclerosis, which might be expected to occur more frequently in the diabetic, appear not to do so (Munichoodappa et al, 1979). However, renal dysfunction, especially in long-standing insulin-dependent diabetes, is the exception, although whether hypertension is the cause or a result of the nephropathy remains uncertain.

Several classifications have been proposed although a modification of that recently advocated (Christlieb, 1982) appears a practical and useful guide for management (Table 3.1).

It is important to subdivide the hypertensive diabetic into insulin-dependent (Type 1) or non-insulin-dependent (Type 2). Each type may have hypertension with or without evidence of nephropathy. The form of the elevated blood pressure may be isolated systolic, isolated diastolic or a combination of both. Although this basic classification will suffice for the vast majority of hypertensive diabetics, it is extremely important to delineate the numerically small percentage of those whose elevated blood pressure is associated with neuropathy as these will present an additional therapeutic challenge.

Several authorities have stated that malignant hypertension (implying the presence of arterial fibrinoid necrosis and usually a diastolic blood

Table 3.1 Practical classification of hypertension associated with diabetes mellitus

---

Insulin-dependent diabetes (Type 1)

Hypertension without nephropathy
    Isolated systolic
    Isolated diastolic
    Combined

Hypertension with nephropathy
    Isolated systolic
    Isolated diastolic
    Combined

Hypertension with neuropathy
    often with supine hypotension

Non-insulin-dependent diabetes (Type 2)

Hypertension without nephropathy
Hypertension with nephropathy

---

pressure >140 mmHg with retinal changes such as haemorrhages, exudates and papilloedema) is rare in diabetics and that generally the degree of hypertension tends not to be severe (Drury, 1983). In a recent study the mean systolic blood pressure of hypertensive diabetics (n=203) was 174±27 mmHg and diastolic blood pressure 89±14 mmHg (Pacy et al, 1985). Similar mean blood-pressure levels were recorded in both those receiving insulin and those on diet with or without oral hypoglycaemic agents, demonstrating that hypertension in the diabetic is not particularly severe.

Pathogenesis of Hypertension

Blood pressure is dependent upon two factors: cardiac output and peripheral resistance. However, the precise role of these in the diabetic hypertensive is not known. Several pathophysiological mechanisms have been implicated including premature atherosclerosis, increased circulating blood volume, a role for insulin, body sodium and catecholamines, abnormal central blood-pressure regulation and abnormalities of function or structure of plasma renin which will now be reviewed.

Premature atherosclerosis

It is now well established that diabetics are prone to early atherosclerosis (Epstein et al, 1965; Pirart, 1978; Kannel & McGee, 1979) which appears no different from that in non-diabetics (Robertson & Strong, 1968). When this occurs in the great blood vessels it may result in loss of the normal damping mechanism of the cardiac output due to the relative inelasticity of these vessels. Clinically the reduced compliance in the great vessels will be manifest as an elevation of the systolic blood pressure, which is perhaps the reason for its frequent occurrence in the diabetic subject (Pacy et al, 1985).

Insulin and sodium

In the non-insulin-dependent diabetic it has been postulated that insulin may play a key role in the pathogenesis of elevated blood pressure. It is now established that insulin has an antinatriuretic action resulting in increased sodium reabsorption probably from the proximal convoluted tubules. It has been shown that only physiological concentrations of insulin c. 30–40 μU/ml are required for such an effect (De Fronzo, 1981). Many non-insulin-dependent subjects are overweight and are therefore likely to be hyperinsulinaemic as a result of insulin resistance. This may result in increased sodium reabsorption with subsequent increased exchangeable body sodium (De Chatel et al, 1977). Indeed, increased exchangeable sodium in diabetics has been reported by one group of research workers who also showed that diuretic therapy lowered blood pressure while reversing the 10 per cent increased exchangeable sodium to normal (De Chatel et al, 1977; Weidmann et al, 1979).

Studies using alloxan-induced diabetes in rats (Christlieb, 1974) and in poorly controlled human diabetics (Christlieb et al, 1975) have suggested that hyperglycaemia *per se* may be associated with increased blood volume (possibly secondary to an osmotic effect of chronic hyperglycaemia). Such an effect along with the antinatriuretic effect of hyperinsulinaemia expands the extracellular compartment at the expense of intracellular dehydration. As long as fluid intake remains adequate to compensate for ensuing polyuria the blood volume will remain expanded with resultant elevation of cardiac output and thus blood pressure.

Renin–angiotensin system

A possible pathological role for the renin–angiotensin system has been proposed. In normotensive and hypertensive diabetics without evidence of nephropathy both raised and normal levels of plasma renin activity have been found (Christleib et al, 1976; De Chatel et al, 1977; Burden & Thursten, 1979). Although studies have revealed that only a small subgroup of such diabetics have reduced plasma renin, in those with nephropathy both plasma renin activity and plasma aldosterone tend to be decreased (Christlieb, 1978). This may be due to a reduction of free water clearance resulting in elevation of the blood volume and suppression of renin while the osmotic effect of hyperglycaemia may further exacerbate the problem. In addition, the physical effect of thickening of the arteriolar walls in the kidney may prevent release of renin from the juxtaglomerular apparatus (Schindler & Sommers, 1966). Defectively synthesized renin (big renin or prorenin) has been shown to have reduced physiological activity (De Leiva et al, 1976). It has also been reported that diabetics may have increased vascular sensitivity to angiotensin II (Christlieb, 1976; Weidmann et al, 1979). This may be important as weight loss with accompanying reduction of blood pressure in obese non-diabetic hypertensives has been shown to be accompanied by reduced levels of plasma renin activity and aldosterone (Tuck et al, 1981).

Catecholamines and the nervous system

Abnormalities of the nervous system have been implicated in the development of hypertension in diabetes. An American report found heart rate to be positively related to blood glucose (Stamler et al, 1975). However, the relationship between blood glucose and blood pressure appeared independent of heart rate and therefore by implication either increased sympathetic activity or parasympathetic denervation. Similar findings were reported in a British study (Jarrett et al 1978). Diabetics have been found to have greater pressor responsiveness than non-diabetics with more pronounced elevation of systolic blood pressure following exercise (Karlefors, 1966). Plasma catecholamine levels tend to be normal in the majority of diabetics except in those with ketoacidosis, autonomic neuropathy and poor glycaemic control (Christensen, 1972; Christlieb, 1976; Zadik et al, 1980), although hypertensive diabetics may have increased sensitivity to circulating catecholamines (Christlieb, 1976; De Chatel et al, 1977).

Obesity

In the non-diabetic there is now considerable data showing a positive relationship between body mass index and blood pressure (Boyle, 1970; Wilcox, 1978; Brennan et al, 1980; Hovell, 1982). The evidence for this statement is based on three separate observations. First, hypertensive subjects tend to increase their weight as the disease progresses (Chiang et al, 1969; Tyroler et al, 1975). Secondly, hypertension is more frequent in obese than non-obese subjects (Paffenbarger et al, 1968; Stamler et al, 1978; Weiss et al, 1978). Lastly, weight loss is frequently accompanied by a reduction in blood pressure (Ramsay et al, 1978; Reisin et al, 1978; Fagerberg et al, 1984; MacMahon et al, 1985).

The pathological mechanisms for this relationship are poorly understood, although several hypotheses have been proposed (Messerli, 1982). Elevated blood pressure itself or antihypertensive therapy may result in an inappropriately high energy intake, and secondly obesity *per se* either due to metabolic changes or consequent upon an increased energy and possibly sodium intake with lack of exercise may predispose an individual to high blood pressure. In addition, it is possible that hypertension and obesity are linked by a common but as yet unknown factor.

Finally this relationship may simply be fictitious, arising from observations with an inappropriately sized sphygmomanometer cuff (Ragan & Bordley, 1941; King, 1967; Maxwell et al, 1982). However, a Belgian study in which cuff width and arm circumference were taken into account revealed that even after correcting for this relationship, weight appeared correlated to blood pressure (Demanet et al, 1976). Many non-insulin-dependent (Type 2) diabetics are overweight and this may be one reason for the high prevalence of hypertension observed in this group. This association, as implied previously, may relate to the antinatriuretic action of insulin which is perhaps the common link between obesity and elevated blood pressure (Bjorntorp, 1982).

Other factors

Several other abnormalities have been described which may be relevant with respect to elevated blood pressure in diabetics. These include increased platelet aggregation and blood viscosity and decreased vascular bed distensibility (Khosla et al, 1979; Faris et al, 1982). In addition, especially in insulin-dependent patients, diabetic nephropathy initially presenting as either overt proteinuria or microalbuminuria may play a key role in the pathogenesis of hypertension.

Is Treatment of Hypertension in Diabetes Beneficial?

There is currently no evidence that adequate antihypertensive therapy in diabetes improves prognosis. However it has been stated that at worst similar results to those in non-diabetics might be anticipated (Christlieb, 1982). In non-diabetics there are now excellent data showing a beneficial effect on several cardiovascular complications by conventional antihypertensive drugs in those with diastolic blood pressure $\geqslant 105\,mmHg$ (Veterans Administration Cooperative Study, 1967, 1979), while the evidence is

conflicting in those with pressures between 90 and 104 mmHg (Kaplan, 1983; Toth & Horwitz 1983) despite claims to the contrary (Hypertension Detection and Follow-up Program Cooperative Group 1979; Australian Therapeutic Trial, 1980). There is no evidence that treating any level of elevated systolic blood pressure is beneficial. It must be borne in mind that the majority of these data have been derived from subjects younger than 65 years (Koch-Weser, 1978) so that the effect of hypotensive drugs in the older age-groups regardless of their blood-pressure status was largely unknown until the recent publication of the European Working Party Trial which did show significant benefits in the elderly (Amery et al, 1985).

Recently there has been speculation that the generally disappointing effects of hypotensive drug therapy in mildly hypertensive subjects may result from the deleterious metabolic side-effects of the agents themselves Multiple Risk Factor Intervention Trial Research Group (1982). In the majority of studies the most frequently used drugs have been thiazide diuretics and beta-blocking agents. Their potentially adverse effects with particular reference to the diabetic will now be outlined.

Adverse Effects of Antihypertensive Agents

Thiazides have been shown to impair carbohydrate, (Lewis et al, 1976; Ames & Hill, 1982; Murphy et al, 1982; Bengtsson et al, 1984), lipid and lipoprotein metabolism (Goldman et al, 1980; Joos et al, 1980; Grimm et al, 1981), and may result in impotence (Report of Medical Research Council Working Party on Mild to Moderate Hypertension, 1981).

Thiazide diuretic agents might adversely influence carbohydrate metabolism in several ways. The importance of potassium depletion has been suggested in several studies (Conn, 1965; Gorden, 1973), and in another potassium supplementation was noted to reverse the detrimental effect on carbohydrate metabolism

(Helderman et al, 1983). In addition, there is some evidence that thiazide diuretic agents reduce tissue sensitivity to insulin (Hicks et al, 1973), accelerate the lack of insulin in the prediabetic subject (Weller & Borondy, 1965) and possibly reduce pancreatic insulin secretion (Shapiro et al, 1961). It has also been reported that frusemide inhibits glucose transport (Jung & Mookerjee, 1976).

A number of mechanisms have been implicated to account for the adverse effect of thiazide diuretics on lipid metabolism, which include reduced lipoprotein lipase activity secondary to the decrease in insulin action (Grimm et al, 1981). Changes in plasma volume may be important (Ames & Hill, 1976), although several observations make this rather unlikely (Tarazi et al, 1970; Joos et al, 1980; Grimm et al, 1981). In addition, thiazide diuretics have been reported to inhibit phosphodiesterase activity (Senft et al, 1966) resulting in elevated cyclic 3, 5-adenosine monophosphate levels which in turn might stimulate lipolysis in fat tissue (Himms-Hagen, 1972).

β-blockers may also adversely influence carbohydrate, lipid and lipoprotein metabolism which appears particularly pronounced with the non-cardioselective agents (Tanaka et al, 1976; Wright et al, 1979; Leren et al, 1980; Day et al, 1982; Veterans Administration Co-operative Study Group on Hypertensive Agents, 1982; Bengtsson et al, 1984). β-blockade might impair carbohydrate metabolism either as a consequence of direct β-adrenoreceptor blockade or as the result of relatively unopposed α activity, either of which might suppress insulin release. Indirect evidence of the latter being important is available from studies of the hyperglycaemic effect of clonidine, an α-adrenergic agonist (Hoefke, 1980). β-blocking agents may adversely influence lipid and lipoprotein levels secondary to α-adrenergic stimulation which may inhibit lipoprotein lipase activity (Day et al, 1982). In addition, catecholamine levels are elevated during β blockade (Rahn et al, 1978) and studies *in vitro* have demonstrated that catecholamines inactivate lipoprotein lipase

(Ashby et al, 1979).

There has been considerable concern about the use of β-blocking drugs in diabetic patients in connection with hypoglycaemia and the peripheral circulation. These drugs may aggravate hypoglycaemia (Newman, 1976; Lager et al, 1979), may result in undamped hypertensive surges secondary to hypoglycaemic catecholamine release (McMurty, 1974; Shepherd et al, 1981) and may threaten the peripheral circulation by arteriolar constriction (McSorley & Warren, 1978; Vale & Jeffreys, 1978). Although symptoms such as tachycardia and tremor are masked, sweating, a predominantly α-mediated response, appears more pronounced during hypoglycaemia with β blockade (Molnar & Read, 1973; Viberti et al, 1978). Despite such theoretical problems, a clinical study found that β-blocking agents were safe in insulin-treated diabetics (Barnett et al, 1980). The adverse effect on the peripheral circulation is probably due to α-mediated vasoconstriction in the blood vessels. In addition, these agents may aggravate cardiac failure, a common complication in the diabetic (Garcia et al, 1974; Kannel & McGee, 1979).

Many of the other hypotensive agents may also have side-effects that may be especially detrimental to the diabetic and these are shown in Table 3.2.

Diet and Blood Pressure

The generally disappointing effects of conventional drug therapy in mild hypertension have resulted in revived interest in non-pharmacological means of lowering blood pressure. In non-diabetics several individual dietary modifications such as diets low in sodium (MacGregor et al, 1982; Hoffman et al, 1983) and fat (Rao et al, 1981; Puska et al, 1983) while high in potassium (Khaw & Thom, 1982; MacGregor et al, 1982) and fibre (Wright et al, 1979; Rouse et al, 1983) have been shown to lower blood pressure.

Exactly how sodium restriction exerts its hypotensive action and why in only certain people remains unknown. It has been observed

Table 3.2 Complications of oral hypotensive drugs with reference to their use in diabetic subjects

Drug	Complications

Thiazide diuretics
Bendrofluazide
	↑ Glucose (Lewis et al, 1976; Ames & Hill, 1982; Murphy et al, 1982;
	    Bengtsson et al, 1984)
	↑ Cholesterol (Goldman et al, 1980; Joos et al, 1980; Grimm et al, 1981)
	↑ Triglyceride (Goldman et al, 1980; Joos et al, 1980; Grimm et al, 1981)
	↑ LDL-cholesterol (Goldman et al, 1980; Joos et al, 1980; Grimm et al, 1981)
	↓ HDL-cholesterol (Gluck et al, 1980)
	Impotence (Report of Medical Research Working Council on Mild to Moderate
	    Hypertension, 1981)

β-adrenergic blockers Cardioselective agents Metoprolol	↑ Glucose (Wright et al, 1979) ↑ Triglyceride (Shaw et al, 1978; Day et al, 1982) ↓ HDL-cholesterol (Day et al, 1982) Aggravate hypoglycaemia (Newman, 1976) Precipitate hypertensive crisis (Shepherd et al, 1981) Precipitate cardiac failure Precipitate intermittent claudication

Non-selective agents
Propranolol
	↑ Glucose (Wright et al, 1979; Gundersen & Kjekshus. 1983;
	    Dornhorst et al, 1985)
	↑ Triglyceride (Lehtonen & Viikari, 1979; Leren et al, 1980)
	↑ Cholesterol (Lehtonen & Viikari, 1979)
	↑ LDL-cholesterol (Lehtonen & Viikari, 1979)
	↓ HDL-cholesterol (Tanaka et al, 1976; Lehtonen & Viikari. 1979;
	    Peden et al, 1984)
	Aggravate hypoglycaemia (Newman, 1976)
	Precipitate hypertensive crisis (McMurty, 1974)
	Precipitate peripheral gangrene (Vale & Jeffreys, 1978)
	Precipitate cardiac failure
	Precipitate intermittent claudication

Calcium antagonists Nifedipine	↑ Glucose (Charles et al, 1981; Bhatnagar et al, 1984)
Sympathetic inhibitors Methyldopa	↑ Triglyceride (Benfield & Hunter, 1982) Postural hypotension Impotence
Vasodilators Hydralazine	? Precipitate angina (Christlieb, 1982)
α-adrenergic blockers Prazosin	Postural hypotension

that sodium restriction tends to be more beneficial in hypertensives who have low plasma renin activity and in whom the aldosterone response to lowering dietary sodium is poor (Vaughan et al, 1973). The reduction of intravascular fluid volume secondary to sodium restriction may be a relevant factor. An effect on the endogenous natriuretic hormone which may influence vascular tone via an effect on cellular ATPase, modifying the sodium content of vascular tissue, may be important (De Wardner & MacGregor, 1980).

Likewise, how potassium may influence blood pressure is not clearly understood. Proposed mechanisms include stimulation of the erythrocyte sodium : potassium pump, alteration in sodium and volume status, effects on plasma renin, neurogenic mechanisms and an influence on the peripheral vasculature (Tannen, 1985).

Lowering total dietary fat while increasing the percentage of polyunsaturated fat is believed to beneficially influence blood pressures via linoleic acid which is increased by such dietary manipulation. Linoleic acid is a precursor of prostaglandin synthesis from arachidonic acid. The resultant prostaglandins may have a natriuretic or renal vasodilatory effect and thereby lower blood pressure (Galli, 1980; Iacono et al, 1981).

Dietary fibre may exert an influence on blood pressure due to several mechanisms. These include an effect on gastric emptying and intestinal transit time, the reduction of intralu-

Table 3.3 Summary of controlled studies of dietary manipulation on blood pressure in non-diabetic subjects

Studies	Diet	Trial design	Patients (no.)	Duration (weeks)	Blood pressure status	Results†
MacGregor et al (1982)	Low sodium	Double-blind placebo cross-over	19	4	Hyper-tensive	↓S by 10 mmHg* ↓D by 6 mmHg*
Watt et al (1983)	Low sodium	Double-blind placebo cross-over	18	4	Normo-tensive	No effect on blood pressure
Silman et al (1983)	Low sodium	Open compared to 'health package'	12	52	Hyper-tensive	↓S by 29 mmHg ↓D by 18 mmHg but no different from general health package
Hofman et al (1983)	Low sodium	Double-blind	231	25	Normo-tensive Infants	↓S by 2 mmHg* compared to normal sodium diet
Richards et al (1984)	Low sodium or high potassium	Cross-over	12	4	Hyper-tensive	No effect on blood pressure
Puska et al (1983)	Low fat (23%) [PS ratio 1:1]	Cross-over	35	6	Normo-tensive	↓S by 9 mmHg* ↓D by 8 mmHg*
MacGregor et al (1982)	High potassium	Double-blind placebo cross-over	23	4	Hyper-tensive	↓S by 8 mmHg* ↓D by 4 mmHg*
Khaw and Thom (1982)	High potassium	Double-blind placebo cross-over	20	2	Normo-tensive	↓S by 1 mmHg ↓D by 2 mmHg*
Rouse et al (1983)	High fibre	Cross-over	38	6	Normo-tensive	↓S by 7 mmHg* ↓D by 3 mmHg*
Beard et al (1982)	Combination	Open	45	12	Hyper-tensives on treatment	↓S by 11 mmHg* ↓D by 6 mmHg* 82% stopped or reduced hypo-tensive drugs
Smith et al (1985)	Low sodium plus high potassium	Double-blind placebo cross-over	20	4	Hyper-tensive	No effect on blood pressure

*Statistically significant.
† ↓, Reduction; S, systolic; D, diastolic.

minal pressure and colonic faecal transit, all of which may alter central blood pressure regulation via afferent nerves from the gastrointestinal tract (Anderson, 1981). The antinatriuretic effect of insulin has also attracted interest (De Fronzo, 1981). High-fibre diets tend to be associated with lower postprandial insulin concentrations than low-fibre diets (Jenkins et al, 1977). Additionally, the effect of fibre on other gastrointestinal hormones such as gastric inhibitory polypeptide, vasoactive intestinal polypeptide and glucagon may be important, probably through their effect on insulin and its antinatriuretic role (Anderson, 1980).

The effects of such diets individually appear small, which raises the possibility that combining several of these factors may have a more substantial effect. Indeed, a non-controlled (Dodson & Humphreys, 1981) and a controlled (Beard et al, 1982) trial have shown such a combined diet does lower blood pressure and, importantly, the quantity of antihypertensive medication required for good blood pressure control. Some of the studies on the effect of dietary manipulation and blood pressure are shown in Table 3.3. It must be stressed that many other dietary components such as calcium, other divalent ions and trace elements may be equally important with respect to blood pressure (McCarron et al, 1982; Saltman, 1983).

These aforementioned studies were in non-diabetic hypertensive subjects but raised the possibility that similar effects might occur in diabetics. Recently there has been a reappraisal of general dietary considerations for diabetics on both sides of the Atlantic (Nuttall, 1980; Nutrition Sub-Committee of the British Diabetic Association's Medical Advisory Committee, 1982). The recommendations currently include an increased quantity of unrefined or complex carbohydrate and cereal fibre with a reduction of total fat and salt. Such a diet somewhat resembles that of the native Ugandan community where hypertension was exceedingly rare (Orr & Gilks, 1931). Application of this diet has produced encouraging results in essential hypertensives (Dodson & Humphreys, 1981). The

Table 3.4 Composition of the modified diet compared to that considered representative of a modern western diet

Components of diet	Modified diet	Modern western diet (UK)
Total energy (kcal)	1600–2100 (6.5–8.6 MJ)	2250 (9.3 MJ)
Fat (% total energy)	25	40
Protein (% total energy)	22	13
Unrefined carbohydrate (% total energy)	50	26
Refined carbohydrate	0–3 (includes alcohol intake)	21
Dietary fibre (g/day)	40–45	20
Sodium (mmol/day)	60–80	180
Potassium (mmol/day)	80–90	80
Sodium : potassium ratio	1 : 1.5	2 : 1

Values for a modern diet in the UK are derived from the National Advisory Commission on Nutrition Education Report (1983) and the Annual Report of the National Food Survey Committee (Ministry of Agriculture, Fisheries & Food, 1979). Reproduced with the permission of the Controller of her Majesty's Stationery Office.

composition of this combination approach diet compared to that considered a 'normal' Western diet is shown in Table 3.4.

In mildly hypertensive non-insulin-dependent patients a recent controlled study using an intended diet shown in Table 3.4 lowered systolic and diastolic blood pressure, improved glycaemic control and reduced weight during a three-month period (Dodson et al, 1984). In addition, this diet lowered serum triglyceride levels, increased HDL_2-cholesterol and in hyperlipidaemic patients lowered serum cholesterol (Pacy et al, 1984c). In an attempt to evaluate the factors possibly responsible for the reduction of blood pressure linear Pearson correlations were determined between changes in blood pressure and several other variables. Positive correlations were observed between a reduction in the urinary sodium : potassium ratio and urinary sodium excretion with systolic ($P<0.001$ and <0.03, respectively) and diastolic blood pressure ($P<0.001$ and <0.01, respectively). Weight loss was positively correlated with only the reduction of systolic blood pressure ($P<0.01$). Multiple regression analysis confirmed that the reduction in the urinary sodium : potassium ratio was most important relating to the decrease of systolic ($P<0.0006$) and diastolic blood pressure ($P<0.001$) (Dodson et al, 1984). Blacks had as beneficial a response to the diet as whites (Pacy et al, 1985), although results in Asians were generally disappointing (Dodson et al, 1983). The blood-pressure-lowering effect of the diet was similar to that of bendrofluazide (10 mg daily), which significantly worsened glycaemic control and tended to elevate total lipid levels in hyperlipidaemic subjects (Pacy et al, 1984a). Likewise, the dietary hypotensive response was comparable to metoprolol (400 mg daily), which was associated with the onset of intermittent claudication and shortness of breath in two of 25 patients. In hyperlipidaemic subjects metoprolol tended to increase serum triglyceride levels (Pacy et al, 1984b).

Compliance with the diet appeared satisfactory from studies in diabetics and non-diabetics over at least three months. In one study analysis of dietary histories in 29 of 50 diabetics revealed that compliance was adequate for unrefined carbohydrate (39 per cent daily energy), fibre (34 g/day) and sodium (100 mmol/day), although dietary fat was higher than intended (33 per cent daily energy) (Pacy et al, 1984c). More long-term data are scarce, but evidence suggests compliance may be maintained for at least four years with good blood pressure control and improved cardiovascular risk in non-diabetics (Dodson et al, 1982, 1985).

Treatment of the Hypertensive Diabetic

The non-insulin-dependent diabetic

In the light of current data for non-insulin-dependent diabetics without evidence of nephropathy and whose diastolic blood pressure is less than 110 mmHg, the high-fibre low-fat and low-sodium diet described earlier appears to be the preferred therapy and should be continued for at least three months. The obese diabetic (Ideal body weight >120 per cent: Metropolitan Life Insurance Company, 1959) must be encouraged to lose weight as this has been found to have a blood-pressure-lowering effect which may or may not be related to concomitant reduction of dietary sodium (Reisin et al, 1978; Tuck et al, 1981; Fagerberg et al, 1984). However, it must be borne in mind that work from the non-diabetic population has suggested that only between 30 and 50 per cent of patients are sodium sensitive (Kawasaki et al, 1978). Therefore it is unlikely that all patients can be expected to respond favourably to such a diet. It would also appear prudent to encourage increased exercise as preliminary work in non-diabetics shows this may have a beneficial effect on blood-pressure levels in hypertensives (Roman et al, 1981). Lastly, as part of general health care, it is extremely important to discourage cigarette smoking.

Should these general measures fail after a minimum three-month period the drug of first choice is probably a cardioselective ß-blocking agent such as atenolol or metoprolol or alternatively a calcium antagonist such as nifedepine. The latter agents may not cause abnormalities of either carbohydrate or lipid metabolism (Donnelly & Harrower, 1980; Faergeman et al, 1984; Rodjmark & Andersson, 1984), despite several case reports (Charles et al, 1981; Bhatnagar et al, 1984), and they may have fewer side-effects than cardioselective ß-blocking drugs. If satisfactory control of hypertension is not achieved with dietary modification and one of these agents, then they can be used in combination. There seems little justification for the use of thiazides in these patients. In those with diastolic pressure over 110 mmHg on repeated measurement the above drug regimen can be initiated concurrently with dietary modification as control of the hypertension is more urgent. Resistant hypertension poses a problem. The recently developed angiotensin-converting enzyme inhibitors, captopril and enalapril, possibly have a place here. They may be effective alone, but there needs to be caution with their introduction, especially enalapril which may cause hypotension when combined with other agents. Choosing a low dose and avoiding volume depletion will minimise this potential risk. If these agents alone are not completely successful, they can be combined with other agents such as diuretics but, once again, perhaps thiazides are best avoided in diabetics and frusemide used as an alternative. We do of course need some good studies on the angiotensin-converting enzyme inhibitors in diabetic patients. Alternatives to these new agents are prazosin which influences pre- and post-load, or hydralazine which influences after-load (Breckenbridge, 1984).

For patients with isolated systolic hypertension perhaps there is only a place for dietary therapy, as although this form of hypertension is associated with increased mortality and morbidity (Kannel et al, 1980), evidence is lacking that drug therapy is beneficial.

It is also worth bearing in mind that data on the benefits of conventional antihypertensive therapy have been derived to a large extent from subjects less than 65 years of age (Koch-Weser, 1978). Thus in both types of diabetes the threshold for commencing conventional drug therapy should be higher in patients over 65 years of age, although benefit has been shown in older non-diabetics in a recent study (Amery et al, 1985).

The insulin-dependent diabetic

In patients without evidence of nephropathy a similar diet and drug regimen can be used and, if there are features of nephropathy, the inexorable decline of renal function may be slowed by good control of hypertension (Mogensen, 1982; Parving et al, 1983). It has been suggested that blood pressure should be controlled at as near normotensive levels as possible to achieve maximal benefit. There are preliminary data showing that high unrefined carbohydrate diets lower serum creatinine levels in those with renal failure so this could be combined with the suggested drug regime (Rivellese et al, 1984). When renal failure supervenes with sodium and water retention contributing significantly to hypertension, then a diuretic may be particularly useful. Again there are advantages in choosing frusemide in preference to a thiazide in view of the increased risk of impotence and lipid abnormalities with the latter. With the decline of renal function it is extremely important to monitor serum electrolytes closely, especially in those on diuretic therapy. Finally there may be a role for either haemodialysis or continuous ambulatory peritoneal dialysis, and cadaveric renal transplantation must not be forgotten, although assessment for such treatment can only be undertaken at a few specialist centres.

In the neuropathic diabetic supine hypertension with accompanying postural hypotension is extremely difficult to treat. Many of these patients will have hypoaldosteronism and in the face of renal sodium loss the diabetic may well be sodium depleted. In this situation low-sodium diets are contraindicated and a mineralocorticoid may be required. Fludrocortisone is often used, although such replacement therapy must be closely monitored to prevent further elevation of the blood pressure. General measures such as the use of elastic tights and elevating the head of the bed to reduce morning postural hypotension may be of benefit. One should attempt to withhold all conventional hypotensive agents for as long as possible as they will tend to exacerbate the postural hypotension. In addition, as the natural history of this extremely distressing condition is to improve with time, considerable counselling and encouragement will be required.

Summary

There is now good evidence that diabetics have higher levels of blood pressure, particularly systolic blood pressure, than age- and sex-matched non-diabetic subjects. Hypertension is prevalent, with systolic hypertension appearing the most frequent in non-insulin-dependent diabetics, possibly reflecting the frequency of obesity in this group. Evidence for increased diastolic hypertension is less strong and is probably related to renal dysfunction. As in the non-diabetic, hypertension is more common in black compared to white and Asian diabetics. It is likely that hypertension adversely affects overall morbidity and mortality in diabetes and has deleterious effects on the more specific diabetic complications. However, only treatment of hypertension in diabetics with nephropathy has been shown to improve prognosis, although this statement is based on very few patients.

High unrefined carbohydrate, high-fibre, low-fat and low-sodium diets may be the initial treatment of the diabetic with mild hypertension in whom thiazide diuretic agents are relatively contraindicated. Cardioselective ß-blocking drugs appear the drugs of choice in the hypertensive diabetic in whom dietary therapy has failed or who has more severe hypertension, although there may be an important role for the calcium antagonists. However, a great deal more work in both the short and long term is required before the most appropriate hypotensive regimen in diabetes mellitus can be formulated.

References

Amery, A., Birkenhager, W., Brixko, P. et al (1985). Mortality and morbidity results from the European Working Party on High Blood Pressure in the Elderly. *Lancet* **i**, 1349–1354.

Ames, R.P. and Hill, P. (1976). Elevation of serum lipids during diuretic therapy of hypertension. *Am J. Med.* **61**, 748–757.

Ames, R.P. and Hill, P. (1982). Improvement of glucose tolerance and lowering of glycohemoglobin and serum lipid concentrations after discontinuation of anti-hypertensive drug therapy. *Circulation* **65**, 899–904.

Anderson, J.W. (1980). Dietary fiber and diabetes. In Spiller, G.A. and Kay, R.M. (eds), *Medical Aspects of Dietary Fiber*, New York, Plenum, pp. 193–221.

Anderson, J.W. (1981). Plant fiber treatment for metabolic diseases. *Spec. Top. Endocrinol. Metab.* **2**, 1–42.

Ashby, P., Parkin, S.M., Walker, K. et al (1979). Hormonal control of adipose tissue lipoprotein activity. *INSERM Symposium* **87**, 149–160.

Australian Therapeutic Trial (1980). Report by the Management Committee. The Australian Therapeutic Trial in mild hypertension. *Lancet* **i**, 1261–1267.

Barnett, A.H., Leslie, D. and Watkins, P.J. (1980). Can insulin-treated diabetics be given beta-adrenergic blocking drugs. *Br. Med. J.* **1**, 976–978.

Barrett-Connor, E., Criqui, M.H., Klauber, M.R. et al (1981). Diabetes and hypertension in a community of older adults. *Am. J. Epidemiol.* **113**, 276–284.

Beard, T.C., Cooke, H.M., Gray, W.R. et al (1982). Randomised controlled trial of a no-added-sodium diet for mild hypertension. *Lancet* **ii**, 455–458.

Bell, E.T. and Clawson, B.J. (1928). Primary (essential) hypertension. *Arch. Pathol.* **5**, 939–1002.

Benfield, G.F. and Hunter, K.R. (1982). Oxprenolol, methyldopa and lipids in diabetes mellitus. *Br. J. Clin. Pharmacol.* **13**, 219–222.

Bengtsson C., Blehmé, G., Lapidus, L. et al (1984). Do antihypertensive drugs precipitate diabetes? *Br. Med. J.* **289**, 1495–1497.

Bhatnagar, S.K., Amin, M.M.A. and Al-Yusuf, A.R. (1984) Diabetogenic effects of nifedipine. *Br. Med. J.* **289**, 19.

Bjorntorp, P. (1982). Hypertension in obesity. *Acta Med. Scand.* **211**, 241–242.

Boyle, E. (1970). Biological patterns in hypertension by race, sex, body weight and skin color. *JAMA* **213**, 1637–1643.

Breckenbridge, A. (1984). The third drug in hypertension. *Br. Med. J.* **289**, 859–860.

Brennan, P.J., Simpson, J.M., Blacket, R.B. et al (1980). The effects of body weight on serum cholesterol, serum triglycerides, serum urate and systolic blood pressure. *Aust. NZ J. Med.* **10**, 15–20.

Burden, A.C. and Thurston, H. (1979). Plasma renin activity in diabetes mellitus. *Clin. Sci.* **56**, 255–259.

Charles, S., Ketelslegers, J-M., Buysschaert, M. et al (1981). Hyperglycaemic effect of nifedipine. *Br. Med. J.* **283**, 19–20.

Chiang, B.N., Perlman, L.V. and Epstein, F.H. (1969). Overweight and hypertension: a review. *Circulation* **39**, 403–421.

Christensen, N.J. (1972). Plasma catecholamines in

long-term diabetics with and without neuropathy and in hypophysectomized subjects. *J. Clin. Invest.* **51**, 779–787.

Christlieb, A.R. (1974). Renin, angiotensin and norepinephrine in alloxan diabetes. *Diabetes* **23**, 962–970.

Christlieb, A.R. (1976). Vascular reactivity to angiotensin II and to norepinephrine in diabetic subjects. *Diabetes* **25**, 268–274.

Christlieb, A.R. (1978). Nephropathy, the renin system and hypertensive vascular disease in diabetes mellitus. *Cardiovas. Med.* **2**, 417–431.

Christlieb, A.R. (1982). The hypertensions of diabetes. *Diabetes Care* **5**, 50–58.

Christlieb, A.R., Assal, J-P., Katsilambros, N. et al (1975). Plasma renin activity and blood volume in uncontrolled diabetes: ketoacidosis, a state of secondary aldosteronism. *Diabetes* **24**, 190–193.

Christlieb, A.R., Kaldany, A. & D'Elia, J.A. (1976). Plasma renin activity and hypertension in diabetes mellitus. *Diabetes* **25**, 969–974.

Christlieb, A.R., Warran, J.H., Krolewski, A.S. et al (1981). Hypertension: the major risk factor in juvenile-onset insulin-dependent diabetics. *Diabetes* **30**, Suppl. 2, 90–96.

Comstock, G.W. (1957). An epidemiologic study of blood pressure levels in a biracial community in the Southern United States. *Am. J. Hyg.* **65**, 271–315.

Conn, J.W. (1965). Hypertension, the potassium ion and impaired carbohydrate tolerance. *N. Engl. J. Med.* **273**, 1135–1143.

Day, J.L., Metcalfe, J. and Simpson, C.N. (1982). Adrenergic mechanisms in control of plasma lipid concentrations. *Br. Med. J.* **284**, 1145–1148.

De Chatel, R., Weidmann, P., Flammer, J. et al (1977). Sodium, renin, aldosterone, catecholamines and blood pressure in diabetes mellitus. *Kidney Int.* **12**, 412–421.

De Fronzo, R.A. (1981). The effect of insulin on renal sodium metabolism. A review with clinical implications. *Diabetologia* **21**, 165–171.

De Leiva, A., Christlieb, A.R., Melby, J.C. et al (1976). Big renin and biosynthesis defect of aldosterone in diabetes mellitus. *N. Engl. J. Med.* **295**, 639–643.

De Wardner, H.E. and MacGregor, G.A. (1980). Dahl's hypothesis that a saluretic substance may be responsible for a sustained use in arterial pressure: its possible role in essential hypertension. *Kidney Int.* **18**, 1–5.

Demanet, J.C., Rorive, G., Samii, K. et al (1976). Effect of weight on prevalence of hypertension and its interaction with the arm circumference: Belgian Hypertension Committee Epidemiology Study. *Clin. Sci. Mol. Med.* **51**, 665s–667s.

Dodson, P.M. and Humphreys, D. (1981). Hypertension and angina. In Trowell, H.C. and Burkitt, D.P. (eds) *Western Diseases: Their Emergence and Prevention*, London, Edward Arnold, pp. 411–420.

Dodson, P.M., Pacy, P.J., Bal, P. et al (1984). A controlled trial of a high fibre, low fat and low sodium diet for mild hypertension in type 2 (non-insulin dependent) diabetic patients. *Diabetologia*, **27**, 522–526.

Dodson, P.M., Pacy, P.J., Beevers, M. et al (1983). The effects of a high fibre, low fat and low sodium dietary regime on diabetic hypertensive patients of different ethnic groups. *Postgrad. Med. J.* **59**, 641–644.

Dodson, P.M., Pacy, P.J., Cox, E.V. (1985). Four year follow-up of the treatment of essential hypertension with a high fibre, low fat and low sodium dietary regimen. *Human Nutr. Clin. Nutr.* **39c**, 213–20.

Dodson, P.M., Pacy, P.J., Ferns, G.A. et al (1982). High-density lipoproteins and high fibre, low fat diets. *Excerpta Med.* **577**, 31–32.

Donnelly, T. and Harrower, A.D.B. (1980). Effect of nifedipine on glucose tolerance and insulin secretion in diabetic and non-diabetic patients. *Curr. Med. Res. Opin.* **6**, 690–693.

Dornhorst, A., Powell, S.H. and Pensky, J. (1985). Aggravation by propranolol of hyperglycaemic effect of hydrochlorothiazide in type II diabetics without alteration of insulin secretion. *Lancet* i, 123–126.

Drury, P.L. (1983). Diabetes and arterial hypertension. *Diabetologia* **24**, 1–9.

Dunn, J.P., Ipsen, J., Elsom, K.O. et al (1970). Risk factors in coronary artery disease, hypertension and diabetes. *Am. J. Med. Sci.* **259**, 309–322.

Elliott, A.R. (1907). A clinical study of blood pressure variations in diabetes and their bearing on the cardiac complications. *JAMA* **49**, 27–30.

Entmacher, P.S., Root, H.F. and Marks, H.H. (1964). Longevity of diabetic patients in recent years. *Diabetes* **13**, 373–377.

Epstein, F.H., Ostrander, L.B., Johnson, B.C. et al (1965). Epidemiological studies of cardiovascular disease in a total community — Tecumseh, Michigan. *Ann. Intern. Med.* **62**, 1170–1185.

Faergeman, O., Meinertz, H. and Hansen, J.F. (1984). Serum lipoproteins after treatment with verapamil for six months. *Acta Med. Scand.* Suppl. 681, 49–51.

Fagerberg, B., Andersson, O.K., Isaksson, B. et al (1984). Blood pressure control during weight reduction in obese hypertensive men: separate effects of sodium and energy restriction. *Br. Med. J.* **1**, 11–14.

Faris, I., Agerskov, K., Henrikmsen, O. et al (1982). Decreased distensibility of a passive vascular bed in diabetes mellitus: an indicator of microangiopathy.

Diabetologia **23**, 411–414.

Florey, C. du V., Uppal, S. and Lowy C. (1976). Relation between blood pressure, weight, and plasma sugar and serum insulin levels in school children aged 9–12 years in Westland, Holland. *Br. Med. J.* **1**, 1368–1371.

Fuller, J.H., Shipley, M.J., Rose, G. et al (1983). Mortality from coronary heart disease and stroke in relation to degrees of glycaemia: the Whitehall Study. *Br. Med. J.* **287**, 867–870.

Galli, C. (1980). Dietary influence on prostaglandin synthesis *Adv. Nutr. Res.* **3**, 95–126.

Garcia, H.M., McNamara, P.M., Gordon, T. et al (1974). Morbidity and mortality in diabetics in the Framingham population. Sixteen year follow-up study. *Diabetes* **23**, 105–111.

Gluck, Z., Weidmann, P., Mordasini, R. et al (1980). Increased serum low-density lipoprotein cholesterol in men treated short-term with diuretic chlorthalidone. *Metabolism* **29**, 240–245.

Goldman, A.I., Steele, B.W., Schnaper, H.W. et al (1980). Serum lipoprotein levels during chlorthalidone therapy. *JAMA* **244**, 1691–1695.

Goodkin, G. (1975). Mortality factors in diabetes. A 20 year mortality study. *J. Occup. Med.* **17**, 716–722.

Gorden, P. (1973). Glucose intolerance and hypokalaemia. *Diabetes* **22**, 544–551.

Grimm, R.H., Leon, A.S., Hunninghake, D.B. et al (1981). Effects of thiazide diuretics on plasma lipids and lipoproteins in mildly hypertensive patients. A double-blind controlled trial. *Ann. Intern. Med.* **94**, 7–11.

Gundersen, T. and Kjekshus, J. (1983). Timolol treatment after myocardial infarction in diabetic patients. *Diabetes Care* **6**, 285–290.

Hawthorne, V.M., Greaves, D.A. & Beevers, D.G. (1974). Blood pressure in a Scottish town. *Br. Med. J.* **3**, 600–603.

Hayward, R.E. and Lucena, B.C. (1965). An investigation into the mortality of diabetics. *J. Instit. Actuar.* **91**, 286–336.

Helderman, J.H., Elahi, D., Andersen, D.K. et al (1983). Prevention of the glucose intolerance of thiazide diuretics by maintenance of body potassium. *Diabetes* **32**, 106–111.

Hicks, B.H., Ward, J.D., Jarrett, R.I. et al (1973). A controlled trial of clopamide, clorexolone and hydrochlorothiazide in diabetics. *Metabolism* **22**, 101–109.

Himms-Hagen, J. (1972). Effects of catecholamines on metabolism. In Blaschko, H. and Muscholl, E. (eds) Berlin, Springer, *Catecholamines (Handbook of Experimental Pharmacology, Vol. 33)*, pp. 363–462.

Hoefke, W. (1980). Clonidine. In Scriabine, A. (ed.) *Pharmacology of Antihypertensive Agents*, New York, Raven Press, PP. 55–78.

Hofman, A., Hazelbroek, A. and Valkenburg, H.A. (1983). A randomised trial of sodium intake and blood pressure in newborn infants. *JAMA* **250**, 370–373.

Hovell, M.F. (1982). The experimental evidence for weight-loss treatment of essential hypertension: a critical review. *Am. J. Public Health* **72**, 359–368.

Hypertension Detection and Follow-up Program Co-operative Group (1977). Blood pressure studies in 14 communities. A two-stage screen for hypertension. *JAMA* **237**, 2385–2391.

Hypertension Detection and Follow-up Program Co-operative Group (1979). Reduction in mortality of persons with high blood pressure including mild hypertension. *JAMA* **242**, 2562–2571.

Iacono, J.M., Judd, J.T., Marshall, M.W. et al (1981). The role of dietary essential fatty acids and prostaglandins in reducing blood pressure. *Prog. Lipid Res.* **20**, 349–364.

Jarrett, R.J., Keen, H., McCartney, M. et al (1978). Glucose tolerance and blood pressure in two population samples: their relation to diabetes mellitus and hypertension. *Int. J. Epidemiol.* **7**, 15–24.

Jenkins, D.J.A., Leeds, A.R., Gassull, M.A. et al (1977). Decrease in post prandial insulin and glucose concentrations by guar and pectin. *Ann. Intern. Med.* **86**, 20–23.

John, H.J. (1932). Hypertension and diabetes. *Ann. Intern. Med.* **5**, 1462–1486.

Joos, C., Kewitz, H. and Reinhold-Kourniati, D. (1980). Effects of diuretics on plasma lipoproteins in healthy man. *Eur. J. Clin. Pharmacol.* **17**, 251–257.

Jung, C.Y. and Mookerjee, B.K. (1976). Inhibitory effect of furosemide on glucose transport. *J. Clin. Lab. Med.* **87**, 960–966.

Kannel, W.B., Dawber, T.R. and McGee, D.L. (1980). Perspectives on systolic hypertension. *Circulation* **61**, 1179–1182.

Kannel, W.B. and McGee, D.L. (1979). Diabetes and glucose tolerance as risk factors for cardiovascular disease. The Framingham study. *Diabetes Care* **2**, 120–126.

Kannel, W.B. and McGee, D.L. (1979). Diabetes and cardiovascular disease: The Framingham Study. *JAMA* **241**, 1225–1229.

Kaplan, N.M. (1983). Mild hypertension. When and how to treat. *Arch. Intern. Med.* **143**, 255–259.

Karlefors, T. (1966). Exercise tests in male diabetics. II. Heart rate and systolic blood pressure. *Acta Med. Scand.* **180**, Suppl., 19–43.

Kawasaki, T., Delea, C.S., Bartter, F.C. et al (1978). The effect of high-sodium and low-sodium intakes on blood pressure and other related variables in human subjects with idiopathic hypertension. *Am. J. Med.* **64**, 193–198.

Keen, H., Track, N.S. and Sowry, G.C. (1975). Arterial pressure in clinically apparent diabetes. *Diabete Metab.* **1**, 159–164.

Kessler, I.I. (1971). Mortality experience of diabetic patients. A twenty-six year follow-up study. *Am. J. Med.* **51**, 715–724.

Keys, A. (1975). Coronary heart disease—the global picture. *Atherosclerosis* **22**, 149–192.

Khaw, K.T. and Thom, S. (1982). Randomised double-blind cross-over trial of potassium on blood pressure in normal subjects. *Lancet* **ii**, 1127–1129.

Khosla, P.K., Mahabaleswara, M. Tiwara, H.K. et al (1979). Platelet aggregation and retinal microangiopathy in diabetes and hypertension. *Acta Haematol.* **61**, 161–167.

King, G.E. (1967). Errors in clinical measurement of blood pressure in obesity. *Clin. Sci.* **32**, 223–237.

Koch-Weser, J. (1978). Arterial hypertension in old age. *Herz*, **3**, 235–244.

Kramer, D.W. (1928). Hypertension and diabetes. *Am. J. Med. Sci* **176**, 23–31.

Lager, I., Blohme, G. and Smith, U. (1979). Effect of cardioselective and non-cardioselective beta-blockade on the hypoglycaemic response in insulin-dependent diabetics. *Lancet* **i**, 458–462.

Lehtonen, A. and Viikari, J. (1979). Long term effect of sotalol on plasma lipids. *Clin. Sci.* **57**, 4055–4075.

Leren, P., Foss, P.O., Helgeland, A. et al (1980). Effects of propranolol and prazosin on blood lipids. *Lancet* **ii**, 4–6.

Lewis, P.J., Kohner, E.M., Petrie, A. et al (1976). Deterioration of glucose tolerance in hypertensive patients on prolonged diuretic treatment. *Lancet* **i**, 564–566.

McCarron, D.A., Henry, H.J. and Morris, C.D. (1982). Human nutrition and blood pressure regulation: an integrated approach. *Hypertension* **4**, suppl. 111, 2–13.

MacGregor, G.A., Markandu, N.D., Best, F.E. et al (1982). Double-blind randomised cross-over trial of moderate sodium restriction in essential hypertension. *Lancet* **i**, 351–355.

MacGregor, G.A., Smith, S.J., Markandu, N.D. et al (1982). Moderate potassium supplementation in essential hypertension. *Lancet* **ii**, 567–570.

MacMahon, S.W., Macdonald, G.J., Bernstein, L. et al (1985). Comparison of weight reduction with metoprolol in treatment of hypertension in young overweight patients. *Lancet* **i**, 1233–1236.

McMurty, R.J. (1974). Propranolol, hypoglycaemia and hypertensive crisis. *Ann. Intern. Med.* **80**, 669–670.

McSorley, P.D. and Warren, D.J. (1978). Effects of propranolol and metoprolol on the peripheral circulation. *Br. Med. J.* **2**, 1598–1600.

Major, S.G. (1929). Blood pressure in diabetes mellitus: a statistical study. *Arch. Intern. Med.* **44**, 797–812.

Marble, A. (1976). Late complications of diabetes. A continuing challenge. *Diabetologia* **12**, 193–199.

Maxwell, M.H., Waks, A.U., Schroth, P.C. et al (1982). Error in blood-pressure measurement due to incorrect cuff size in obese patients. *Lancet* **ii**, 33–36.

Messerli, F.H. (1982). Cardiovascular effects of obesity and hypertension. *Lancet* **i**, 1165–1168.

Metropolitan Life Insurance Company (1959). New weight standards for men and women. *Stat. Bull.* **40**, 1–10.

Miller, N.E., Hammett, F., Saltissi, S. et al (1981). Relation of angiographically defined coronary artery disease to plasma lipoprotein subfractions and apolipoproteins. *Br. Med. J.* **282**, 1741–1744.

Ministry of Agriculture, Fisheries and Food (1979). *Household Food Consumption and Expenditure*, London, Her Majesty's Stationery Office, p. 111.

Mogensen, C.E. (1982). Long-term antihypertensive treatment inhibiting progression of diabetic nephropathy. *Br. Med. J.* **285**, 685–686.

Molnar, G.W. and Read, R.C. (1973). Propranolol enhancement of hypoglycemic sweating. *Clin. Pharmacol. Ther.* **15**, 490–496.

Moss, A.J. (1962). Blood pressure in children with diabetes mellitus. *Paediatrics* **30**, 932–936.

Multiple Risk Factor Intervention Trial Research Group (1982). Multiple Risk Factor Intervention Trial. Risk factor changes and mortality results. *JAMA* **248**, 1465–1477.

Munichoodappa, C., D'Elia, J.A., Libertino, J.A. et al (1979). Renal artery stenosis in hypertensive diabetics. *J. Urol.* **121**, 555–558.

Murphy, M.B., Lewis, P.J., Kohner, E. et al (1982). Glucose intolerance in hypertensive patients treated with diuretics: a fourteen year follow-up *Lancet* **ii**, 1293–1295.

National Advisory Committee on Nutrition Education (1983). Proposals for nutritional guidelines for health education in Britain. *Lancet* **ii**, 719–721, 782–785, 835–837, 902–905.

Newman, R.J. (1976). Comparison of propranolol, metoprolol and acebutolol on insulin-induced hypoglycaemia. *Br. Med. J.* **2**, 447–449.

Nutrition Sub-committee of the British Diabetic Association's Medical Advisory Committee (1982). Dietary recommendations for the 1980s—a policy statement by the British Diabetic Association. *Hum. Nutr. Appl. Nutr.* **36**, 378–386.

Nuttall, F.Q. (1980). Dietary recommendations for individuals with diabetes mellitus, 1979: Summary of report from the Food and Nutrition Committee of the American Diabetes Association. *Am. J. Clin. Nutr.* **33**, 1311–1312.

Orr, J.B. and Gilks, J.L. (1931). The physique and

health of two African tribes. *Med. Res. Counc. Spec. Rep. Ser.* **155**, 15–66.

Ostrander, L.D. Jr, Francis, T. Jr, Hayner, N.S. et al (1965). The relationship of cardiovascular disease to hyperglycaemia. *Ann. Intern. Med.* **62**, 1188–1198.

Pacy, P.J., Dodson, P.M., Beevers, M. et al (1985). Prevalence of hypertension in white, black and asian diabetics in a district hospital diabetic clinic. *Diabetic Med.* **2**, 125–130.

Pacy, P.J., Dodson, P.M., Kubicki, A.J. et al (1984 a). Comparison of the hypotensive and metabolic effects of bendrofluazide therapy and a high fibre low fat low sodium diet on diabetic subjects with mild hypertension. *J. Hypert.* **2**, 215–220.

Pacy, P.J., Dodson, P.M., Kubicki, A.J. et al (1984 b). Comparison of the hypotensive and metabolic effects of metoprolol therapy with a high fibre, low sodium, low fat diet in hypertensive type II diabetic subjects. *Diabetes Res.* **1**, 201–207.

Pacy, P.J., Dodson, P.M., Kubicki, A.J. et al (1984 c). Effect of a high fibre high carbohydrate dietary regimen on serum lipids and lipoprotein in type II hypertensive diabetic patients. *Diabetes Res.* **1**, 159–163.

Pacy, P.J., Dodson, P.M., Webster, J. et al (1985). Effect of a high fibre, low fat and low sodium diet in white European and West Indian black type II diabetic patients with mild hypertension. *Proc. Nutr. Soc.* **44**, 69A.

Paffenbarger, R.S., Rhorna, M.C. and Wing, S.L. (1968). Chronic disease in former college students. VIII Characteristics in youth predisposing to hypertension in later years. *Am. J. Epidemiol.* **88**, 25–30.

Parving, H.H., Andersen, A.R., Smidt, U.M. et al (1983). Early aggressive antihypertensive treatment reduces rate of decline in kidney function in diabetic nephropathy. *Lancet* i, 1175–1179.

Peden, N.R., Dow, R.J., Isles, T.E. et al (1984). β Adrenoceptor blockade and responses of serum lipids to a meal and to exercise. *Br. Med. J.* **288**, 1788–1790.

Pell, S. and D'Alonzo, C.A. (1967). Some aspects of hypertension in diabetes mellitus. *JAMA* **202**, 104–110.

Pell, S. & D'Alonzo, C.A. (1970). Factors associated with long-term survival of diabetics. *JAMA* **214**, 1833–1840.

Pirart, J. (1978). Diabetes mellitus and its degenerative complications: a prospective study of 4,400 patients observed between 1947–1973. *Diabetes Care* **1**, 168–188, 252–263.

Puska, P., Iacono, J.M., Nissinen, A. et al (1983). Controlled randomised trial of the effect of dietary fat on blood pressure. *Lancet* i, 1–5.

Ragan, C. and Bordley, J. (1941). The accuracy of clinical measurements of arterial blood pressure. *Bull. J. Hop. Hosp.* **69**, 504–527.

Rahn, K.H., Gierlichs, W., Planz, G. et al (1978). Studies on the effects of propranolol on plasma catecholamine levels in patients with essential hypertension. *Eur. J. Clin. Invest.* **8**, 143–148.

Ramsay, L.E., Ramsay, M.H., Hettiarachchi, J. et al (1978). Weight reduction in a blood pressure clinic. *Br. Med. J.* **2**, 244–245.

Rao, R.H., Rao, U.B. and Srikantia, S.G. (1981) Effect of polyunsaturated-rich vegetable oils on blood pressure in essential hypertension. *Clin. Exp. Hypert.* **3**, (1), 27–38.

Reisin, E., Abel, R., Modan, M. et al (1978). Effect of weight loss without salt restriction on the reduction of blood pressure in overweight hypertensive patients. *N. Engl. J. Med.* **298**, 1–6.

Report of Medical Research Council Working Party on mild to moderate hypertension (1981). Adverse reactions to bendrofluazide and propranolol for the treatment of mild hypertension. *Lancet* ii, 539–543.

Richards, A.M., Nicholls, M.G., Espiner, E.A. et al (1984). Blood-pressure response to moderate sodium restriction and to potassium supplementation in mild essential hypertension. *Lancet* i, 757–761.

Rivellese, A., Parille, M., Perrotti, N. et al (1984). High fibre diets: a useful approach for the treatment of diabetic patients with chronic renal failure. *Abstract Book of the 2nd International Symposium on Diabetes and Nutrition. Dusseldorf 1984.*

Robertson, W.B. and Strong, J.P. (1968). Atherosclerosis in persons with hypertension and diabetes mellitus. *Lab. Invest.* **18**, 538–551.

Rodjmark, S. and Andersson, D.E.H. (1984). Influence of verapamil on glucose tolerance. *Acta Med. Scand.* Suppl. 681, 37–42.

Roman, O., Camuzzi, A.L., Villalon, E. et al (1981). Physical training program in arterial hypertension. *Cardiology* 67, 230–243.

Rouse, I.L., Beilin, L.J., Armstrong, B.K. et al (1983). Blood pressure lowering effect of a vegetarian diet: controlled trial in normotensive subjects. *Lancet* i, 5–9.

Saltman, P. (1983). Trace elements and blood pressure. *Ann. Intern. Med.* **98**, (Part 2), 823–827.

Schindler, A.M. and Sommers, S.C. (1966). Diabetic sclerosis of the renal juxtaglomerular apparatus. *Lab. Invest.* **15**, 877–884.

Senft, G., Losert, W., Schultz, G. et al (1966). Ursachen der storungen im kohlenhydratestoffwechsel unter dem eim fluk sulfonamidierter diuretica. Naunyn-Schmiedebergs *Arch. Pharmak. Exp. Pathol.* **255**, 369–382.

Shapiro, A.P., Benedek, T.G. and Small, J.L. (1961). Effect of thiazides on carbohydrate metabolism in patients with hypertension. *N. Engl. J. Med.* **265**, 1028–1033.

Shaw, J., England, J.D.F. and Hua, A.S.P. (1978). Beta-blockers and plasma triglycerides. *Br. Med. J.* **1**, 986.

Shepherd, A.M.M., Lin, M-S. and Keeton, T.K. (1981). Hypoglycaemia induced hypertension in a diabetic patient on metoprolol. *Ann. Intern. Med.* **94**, 357–358.

Sherrill, J.W. (1933). Cardiovascular disease in diabetes mellitus. An analysis of four hundred and twenty-five cases. *Calif. West Med.* **38**, 73–78.

Silman, A.J., Locke, C., Mitchell, P. et al (1983). Evaluation of a low sodium diet in the treatment of mild to moderate hyerptension. *Lancet* **i**, 1179–1182.

Sive, P.H., Medalie, J.H., Kahn, H.A. et al (1971). Distribution and multiple regression analysis of blood pressure in 10,000 Israeli men. *Am. J. Epidemiol.* **93**, 317–327.

Smith, S.J., Markandu, N.D., Sagnella, G.A. et al (1985). Moderate potassium chloride supplementation in essential hypertension: is it additive to moderate sodium restriction. *Br. Med. J.* **290**, 110–113.

Stamler, J., Rhomberg, P., Schoenberger, J.A. et al (1975). Multivariate analysis of the relationship of seven variables to blood pressure. *J. Chronic Dis.* **28**, 527–548.

Stamler, R., Stamler, J.,Riedlinger, W.F. et al (1978). Weight and blood pressure: findings in hypertension screening of 1 million Americans. *JAMA* **240**, 1607–1612.

Tanaka, N., Sakaguchi, S., Oshige, K. et al (1976). Effect of chronic administration of propranolol on lipoprotein composition. *Metabolism* **25**, 1071–1075.

Tannen, R.L. (1983). Effects of potassium on blood pressure control. *Ann. Intern. Med.* **93**, (Part 2), 773–780.

Tarazi, R.C., Dunstan, H.P. and Frohlich, E.D. (1970). Long term thiazide therapy in essential hypertension. *Circulation* **41**, 708–717.

Toth, P.J. and Horwitz, R.I. (1983). Conflicting clinical trials and the uncertainty of treating mild hypertension. *Am. J. Med.* **75**, 482–488.

Tuck, M.L., Sowers, J., Dornfeld, L. et al (1981). The effect of weight reduction on blood pressure, plasma renin activity and plasma aldosterone levels in obese patients. *N. Engl. J. Med.* **304**, 930–933.

Tunbridge, W.M.G. (1981). Factors contributing to deaths of diabetics under fifty years of age. *Lancet* **ii**, 569–572.

Tyroler, H.A., Heyden, S. and Hames, C.G. (1975). Weight and hypertension: Evans County studies of Blacks and Whites. In Paul, O. (ed.) *Epidemiology and Control of Hypertension*, New York, Stratton Intercontinental, pp. 177–201.

Vale, J.A. and Jeffreys, D.B. (1978). Peripheral gangrene complicating beta-blockade. *Lancet* **i**, 1216.

Vaughan, E.D. Jr, Laragh, J.H., Gavras, I. et al (1973). Volume factor in low and normal renin essential hypertension: treatment with either spironolactone or chlorthalidone. *Am. J. Cardiol.* **32**, 523–532.

Veterans Administration Co-operative Study (1967). Effects of treatment on morbidity in hypertension: results in patients with diastolic blood pressure averaging 115 through 129 mmHg. *JAMA* **202**, 1028–1034.

Veterans Administration Co-operative Study (1979). Effects of treatment on morbidity in hypertension II. Results in patients with diastolic blood pressure averging 90 through 114 mmHg. *JAMA* **213**, 1143–1152.

Veterans Administration Co-operative Study Group on Antihypertensive Agents (1982). Comparison of propranolol and hydrochlorothiazide for the initial treatment of hypertension. II. Results of long-term therapy. *JAMA* **248**, 2004–2011.

Viberti, G.C., Stimmler, H. and Keen, H. (1978). The effect of oxprenolol on the hypoglycaemic response to insulin in normals and insulin-depedent diabetics. *Diabetologia* **15**, 278.

Watt, G.C.M., Edwards, C., Hart, J.T. et al (1983). Dietary sodium restriction for mild hypertension in general practice. *Br. Med. J.* **286**, 432–436.

Weidmann, P., Beretta-Piccoli, C., Kensch, G. et al (1979). Sodium-volume factor, cardiovascular reactivity and hypotensive mechanism of diuretic therapy in mild hypertension associated with diabetes mellitus. *Am. J. Med.* **67**, 779–784.

Weiss, Y.A., Safar, M.E., London, G.M. et al (1978). Repeat hemodynamic determinations in borderline hypertension. *Am. J. Med.* **64**, 382–387.

Weller, J.M. and Borondy, P.E. (1965). Effects of benzothiadazine drugs on carbohydrate metabolism. *Metabolism* **14**, 708–714.

Wilcox, R. (1978). Serum lipid concentrations and blood pressure in obese women. *Br. Med. J.* **1**, 1513–1515.

World Health Organisation (1979). *Report of a WHO Expert Committee on Hypertension*, Geneva, WHO Technical Report Series.

Wright, A., Burstyn, P.G. and Gibney, M.J. (1979). Dietary fibre and blood pressure. *Br. Med. J.* **2**, 1541–1543.

Wright, A.D., Barber, S.G., Kendall, M.J. et al (1979). Beta-adrenoreceptor-blocking drugs and blood sugar control in diabetes mellitus. *Br. Med. J.* **1**,

159–161.

Zadik, Z., Kayne, R., Kappy, M. et al (1980). Increased integrated concentration of norepinephrine, epinephrine, aldosterone and growth hormone in patients with uncontrolled juvenile diabetes mellitus. *Diabetes* **29**, 655–658.

Chapter Four

Lipids, Lipoproteins and Diabetes Mellitus

P.M. Dodson

Dr Paul M. Dodson qualified at St. Bartholomew's Hospital, London, in 1974. He spent his early years in training at Southampton General Hospital and the Royal Berkshire Hospital, Reading. He returned to St Bartholomew's and Moorfields Eye Hospital, London, in 1979 to research hyperlipidaemias that led to his MD. He moved to Dudley Road Hospital, Birmingham, as Senior Registrar in Medicine and Diabetes in 1982 and his current research interests include nutrition in hypertension, diabetes mellitus, lipid metabolism and retinovascular disease.

Introduction

Although microvascular disease is the specific lesion usually associated with diabetes mellitus, atherosclerosis, particularly of the coronary vessels, accounts for the major morbidity and mortality in diabetic patients. The evidence for this is derived from reported clinical and autopsy data in which macrovascular disease accounts for about 75 per cent of all deaths in diabetics, compared to approximately 50 per cent in the non-diabetic population (Ganda, 1980).

Atherosclerosis appears to proceed at a more rapid rate and is more extensive in the diabetic (Crall & Roberts, 1978), but the process does not differ in its morphological appearance nor in its anatomical distribution compared to the non-diabetic (Strandness et al, 1964; Robertson & Strong, 1968). This may be of considerable importance, for in the non-diabetic there are long-established relationships between lipid and lipoprotein levels and macrovascular disease (Gordon et al, 1981; Miller et al, 1981). Similar relationships may be of equal importance in the diabetic subject.

This chapter will therefore examine the relationships between serum lipids and vascular disease in the non-diabetic and the diabetic, together with an outline of lipid metabolism in diabetic patients. Other factors well known to have a prominent effect on serum lipid levels, for example, obesity, diabetic control, drug therapy, alcohol consumption and diet, will be discussed.

Lipid Metabolism

The major large lipid molecules of plasma — triglycerides, cholesterol, cholesterol esters and phospholipids — are predominantly transported by stable complex water-soluble macromolecules, designated lipoproteins. These are made up of a core of non-polar lipids (triglyceride and cholesterol esters) with polar lipids (phospholipids, free cholesterol and apoproteins) located on the outer part of the macromolecules (Galton, et al, 1982).

Free fatty acids, which are bound to albumin, are quantitatively less important than the lipoproteins but may be very significant in the context of poorly controlled diabetes with accumulation and production of ketone bodies.

The main classes of lipoprotein which can be identified by ultracentrifugation are chylomicra, very low density lipoprotein (VLDL), low density lipoprotein (LDL), intermediate density lipoprotein (IDL) and high density lipoprotein (HDL). The composition of these are shown in Table 4.1. The apoprotein components of the lipoproteins are also demonstrated in view of the recent realisation of their importance in lipid metabolism.

Figure 4.1 shows a scheme of the metabolism of lipoproteins and the important regulatory enzymes. The main triglyceride-carrying lipoproteins are secreted by the small intestine and liver as exogenous chylomicra and endogenous VLDL. These are delipidated in peripheral tissues principally by the action of lipoprotein lipase which is secreted by adipose and muscle tissues and attached to the capillary endothelium. Important constituents of VLDL and chylomicra are three apolipoproteins, namely, apo- C II, C III 1 and C III 2, which may be either inhibitory (C III 1 and C III 2) or an obligate activator (C II) of lipoprotein lipase (Galton et al, 1982). Degradation of VLDL produces remnant particles (IDL) which undergo further delipidation to yield LDL. LDL, the major cholesterol-containing lipoprotein, is therefore almost exclusively derived from endogenous metabolism of VLDL. LDL is catabolised by peripheral tissues containing high-affinity cell-surface receptors which bind this lipoprotein, the specificity probably directed to the apo-B component of LDL (Goldstein and Brown, 1974). This process is followed by endocytosis and lysosomal breakdown of LDL. Exogenous cholesterol released inside the cell represses 3-hydroxy 3-methyl glutaryl co-enzyme A (HMG/COA) reductase and there is an increase in the intracellular esterification of cholesterol

Table 4.1 Major lipoprotein classes: composition and physical characteristics

Lipoprotein class	Diameter (A)	Electrophoretic mobility	Major lipid components	Major apolipoprotein present
Chylomicrons	80–500	Origin	Exogenous triglyceride	A I, A II, B, C II, C III
VLDL	30–80	Pre-beta	Triglyceride Cholesterol esters Phospholipid	B, C II, C III
IDL (remnants)	25–35	Slow Pre-beta	Cholesterol esters Triglyceride Phospholipid	B, C III
LDL	18–28	Beta	Cholesterol esters Phospholipid	B
HDL$_2$	10	Alpha	Phospholipid Cholesterol esters	A I, A II, C III
HDL$_3$	7.5	Alpha	Phospholipid Cholesterol esters	A I, A II, C III

Adapted from Jackson et al (1976).
VLDL, very low density lipoprotein; IDL, intermediate density lipoprotein; LDL, low density lipoprotein; HDL, high density lipoprotein (subfractions 2 and 3).

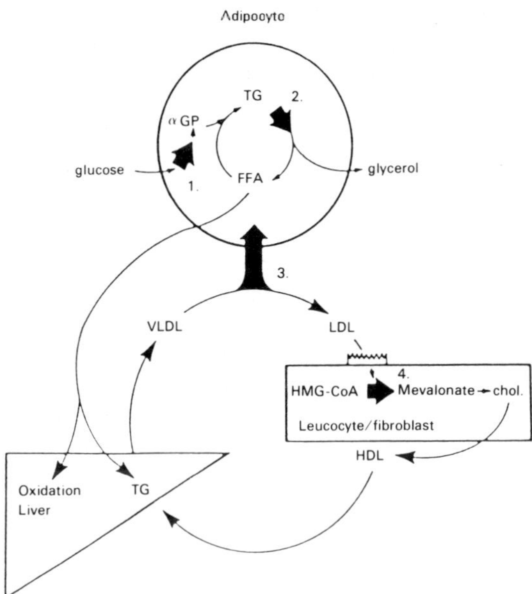

Figure 4.1. A scheme for the metabolism of lipro-
proteins and some of their regulatory enzymes.
Abbreviations: TG, triglyceride; FFA, free fatty acid;
VLDL, very low density lipoprotein; LDL, low
density lipoprotein; HDL, high density lipoprotein;
αGP, *sn*-glycerol 3-phosphate. Regulatory enzymes: 1,
hexokinase-phosphofructokinase; 2, hormone-sensi-
tive triglyceride lipase; 3, lipoprotein lipase; 4, 3-
hydroxy 3-methyl glutaryl coenzyme A reductase.
Figure adapted from that of Galton et al (1982).
Reproduced by permission of John Wiley.

(Goldstein and Brown, 1977). This supply of
cholesterol to the cell by LDL produces feedback
inhibition of intracellular cholesterol synthesis
by repression of the rate-limiting enzyme.
During the breakdown of triglyceride-rich lipoproteins in plasma, the C-apoproteins are lost
from the particle and associate with HDL which
may act as a reservoir for them.

HDL is mainly synthesised in the intestine and
liver. HDL of hepatic origin is secreted as a
discoidal particle containing mostly phospholipids. The discoidal HDL picks up free cholesterol from the cell membranes and, possibly,
from remnant particles and LDL. The lecithin
cholesterol acyl transferase (LCAT) system is
active in this process and generates cholesterol
esters in the HDL and converts them into a

spherical shape. A mature spherical HDL
particle is thus formed after acquiring apo-A
particles from intestinal HDL. Therefore, HDL
may be responsible for the return of cholesterol
from the periphery to the liver where mature
HDL particles are recognised by hepatocyte receptors, leading to uptake and finally degradation for biliary excretion of cholesterol (Tall &
Small, 1978). There are at least two major subfractions of mature HDL, HDL$_2$ and HDL$_3$. It is
thought that the small cholesteryl ester-poor
HDL$_3$ particles are converted to HDL$_2$ as they
acquire cholesterol and later apolipoprotein E,
and that it is the HDL$_2$ which may release cholesterol in the liver (Rothblat & Phillips, 1982;
Gordon et al, 1983). It is also possible that apoproteins and phospholipids resulting from the
breakdown of VLDL to LDL transfer to HDL$_3$
to form a particle resembling HDL$_2$ (Patsch et al,
1978; Tall, 1979).

A description will now be given of the
aetiological theories and relationships that lipids
and lipoprotein levels may have with atherosclerosis.

Lipids and Atherosclerosis

The pathognomonic lesion of atherosclerosis is
the fibrous plaque which is probably due to
proliferation of the smooth muscle cell in the
arterial wall following an initial breach in the
arterial intima (Ross & Glomset, 1976; Ross &
Marker, 1976). This event, according to Ross and
co-workers, is followed by deposition of intracellular and extracellular lipid and accumulation
of other components, including collagen (Ross &
Glomset, 1976; Ross & Marker, 1976).

The exact cause of the initial breach in the
intima is still not identified. The disruption of the
endothelial barriers occurs experimentally with
most forms of injury, including chemical,
mechanical and immune. Several theories of the
factors causing smooth muscle cell proliferation
have been made. These include decline of the
negative feedback of ageing stem cells of the
arterial media thus allowing more rapid replication (Martin et al, 1975; Haylick, 1976), and an as

yet unidentified platelet factor formed during the platelet-release reaction (Ganda, 1980). Finally, LDL has been implicated both as a factor responsible for the initial breach and in the increased smooth muscle cell proliferation (Ross & Marker, 1976; Small, 1977).

The suggestion that LDL may be having a primary effect is supported by the finding of premature atherosclerosis in the presence of most primary hyperlipidaemia, in particular familial hypercholesterolaemia, in which elevated LDL levels are characteristically found. Other evidence suggesting that LDL is important is that LDL enters the arterial intima from plasma at rates directly related to its plasma concentration (Niehaus et al, 1977; Nicoll et al, 1981) and accumulates particularly in atheromatous regions (Nicoll et al, 1981). Endothelial injury increases this process and in some experiments can even be initiated by raised serum lipids, including LDL (Ross & Marker, 1976). Other direct mechanisms may also be operative, as the response of platelets to aggregating agents is enhanced in the presence of media rich cholesterol (Shattil et al, 1975), and might promote thrombotic processes underlying atherosclerosis.

However, other compelling evidence that serum lipids and lipoproteins are causal or primary in the development of atherosclerosis derives from prospective clinical studies in the non-diabetic population and these will be described briefly.

Many studies have shown a relationship between serum cholesterol levels and ischaemic heart disease (Keys, 1970; Kannel et al, 1971; Wilhelmsen et al, 1973; Rosenman et al, 1976; Kannel et al, 1979), and this relationship holds even within the normal range of serum cholesterol concentration. This is well demonstrated in the 14-year prospective Framingham Study, for individuals younger than 50 years the risk of coronary heart disease increased over 5-fold with increasing serum cholesterol levels from 4.6–8.7 mmol/l (Kannel et al, 1979). Other reports have demonstrated an even stronger positive association with plasma LDL choles-

terol which is the main cholesterol-carrying lipoprotein (Castelli et al, 1977; Gordon et al, 1977b). A further test of the hypothesis that increased serum cholesterol and LDL levels are causative is that cholesterol lowering should reduce the incidence of ischaemic heart disease. The recent Lipid Research Clinics primary prevention programme (Lipid Research Clinics Program, 1984), in support of other studies (Dayton et al, 1969; Committee of Principal Investigators, 1978) has demonstrated a significant reduction in the incidence of all coronary artery disease events among patients in whom serum cholesterol was effectively reduced using a combination of diet and cholestyramine.

In contrast, levels of HDL tend to show an inverse relationship with the incidence of coronary artery disease, and hence the name, the protective lipoprotein (Castelli et al, 1977; Gordon et al, 1977b; Miller et al, 1977a). The mechanism of the protective function may be as follows: cholesterol is mobilised from the arterial wall by HDL_3 which is converted to HDL_2 by this process of cholesterol enrichment. Another aspect of the protective function for HDL is possibly reduction of LDL uptake by competitive binding with the LDL receptor, thereby reducing the cholesterol supply to the endothelial cell (Miller et al, 1977 b). These associations have also been confirmed in angiographic studies, as the severity of coronary artery disease increases with increasing LDL and with decreasing HDL levels (Tan et al, 1980; Miller et al, 1981). The protective effect of HDL against atheroma formation is believed to be due to the HDL_2 subfraction (Miller et al, 1981).

The role of serum triglyceride remains controversial. Several studies have reported a positive association with ischaemic heart disease, but after correction for the effect of cholesterol serum triglyceride does not appear to be an independent risk factor (Hulley et al, 1980). Also, these studies did not take into account HDL levels, which are well known to be inversely related to serum triglyceride concentrations (Hulley et al, 1980).

Another site of damage in diabetes may be the

microcirculation which might be important in disease of the myocardium in diabetic subjects. Little data are currently available on serum lipid and lipoprotein levels in relation to microvascular disease, although recent studies in microcirculation in sites other than the myocardium suggest that hyperlipidaemia and increasing LDL levels may be implicated (Dodson et al, 1981 a, 1982).

There are abundant data to support causal associations between serum cholesterol and LDL with macrovascular disease in the non-diabetic (Lewis, 1983). In view of the similarity of atherogenesis in the diabetic and non-diabetic (Strandness et al, 1964; Robertson & Strong, 1968) it is likely that similar relationships apply in diabetic subjects, although the evidence that this is true is not so strong.

Lipid Levels in Diabetes Mellitus

A number of studies have reported that hypertri-

glyceridaemia and hypercholesterolaemia are common in diabetes mellitus. A summary of the major abnormalities of circulating lipid and lipoproteins found according to the type of diabetes are shown in Table 4.2. Despite extensive research, the exact prevalence of hyperlipidaemia has not been determined due to methodological differences. The major problems include the definition of the normal range for fasting cholesterol and triglyceride, failure to divide diabetics into appropriate insulin- or non-insulin-dependent categories, and also the inclusion of newly diagnosed diabetics together with those with long-established disease.

Albrink stated that "hypertriglyceridaemia is the hyperlipidaemia *par excellence* of the diabetic" (Albrink, 1974). Most studies support this statement with prevalence rates for hypertriglyceridaemia ranging from 20–50 per cent, (New et al, 1963; Wilson et al, 1970b; Hayes, 1972; Albrink, 1974; Garcia et al, 1974; Kaufman et al; 1975; Chase & Glasgow, 1976; Nikkila &

Table 4.2 Major abnormalities in circulating lipids found in poorly controlled or newly diagnosed diabetics

| | *Major abnormality* | |
	Type 1 diabetes	*Type 2 diabetes*
Lipids	Hypertriglyceridaemia Hypercholesterolaemia	Hypertriglyceridaemia Hypercholesterolaemia
Lipoproteins	Increased LDL Increased VLDL Increased LDL-triglyceride Normal or elevated HDL	Increased LDL Increased VLDL Increased VDL-triglyceride Normal or reduced HDL
Defects: Triglyceride	Decreased triglyceride clearance Decreased LPL activity with insulin deficiency	Increased endogenous VLDL production Decreased VLDL clearance C-Apolipoprotein defects
Cholesterol	Reduction of LDL receptor numbers in insulin deficiency	An underlying primary genetic hypertri- glyceridaemia commonly present

Increased LDL turnover
Increased LDL synthesis
Non-enzymic glycosylation of LDL altering receptor binding

VLDL, very low density lipoprotein; IDL, intermediate density lipoprotein; LDL, low density lipoprotein; HDL, high density lipoprotein (subfractions 2 and 3).

Hormila, 1978; Mancini et al, 1980; Lisch & Sailer, 1981; Pacy et al, 1985), depending on type of diabetes, diabetic control, age, sex, ethnic origin and nutritional status (in particular, fat and alcohol intake). For example, in the large Framingham population (Garcia et al, 1974), 239 diabetics, of equal sex distribution and age range 30–62 years, were studied prospectively. Thirty-nine per cent of these were insulin treated, 39 per cent were managed on oral hypoglycaemic agents and 22 per cent were not receiving treatment or following a diabetic diet. In this group, 38 per cent of males and 27 per cent of females demonstrated hypertriglyceridaemia. Interestingly, a more marked sex difference was noted for hypercholesterolaemia with prevalence rates in females at 48 per cent and in males 28 per cent. All these prevalence rates were strikingly increased when compared to matched non-diabetic controls except that of hypercholesterolaemia in males. Similar findings to these have also been reported in true Type 1 (insulin-dependent) diabetes (Kaufman et al, 1975).

One recent study has also defined the types of hyperlipidaemia by ultracentrifugation and classified according to the Fredrickson types in a group of 86 Type 2 diabetics and a control group. (Mancini et al, 1980). Hypertriglyceridaemia was well represented with a marked increase in Type 2b, the type with combined hyperlipidaemia, at 24 per cent compared to 2 per cent in the control group. Type 4 hyperlipidaemia, representing mainly hypertriglyceridaemia, was also increased at 18 per cent in the diabetics compared to 10 per cent in controls. Although other types of hyperlipidaemia were not identified in this study, primary hyperlipidaemia, for example, Type 5 characterised by gross increase of the triglyceride-rich lipoprotein, are well documented to occur with diabetes mellitus (Bagdade et al, 1967; Glueck, 1977). Other primary familial hyperlipidaemias may also occur (Brunzell et al, 1975).

The prevalence rate of hypercholesterolaemia in diabetics has been reported to be similar to the non-diabetic population, that is from 8 per cent to as high as 52 per cent (Hayes, 1972).

However, in the majority of studies a high prevalence rate of hypercholesterolaemia has been found (New et al, 1963; Wilson et al, 1970b; Chase & Glasgow, 1976; Mancini et al, 1980; Sosenko et al, 1980; Yano et al, 1982; Pacy et al, 1985). Clinical factors relating to hypercholesterolaemia are similar to those for hypertriglyceridaemia and include obesity, poor diabetic control, increasing age, sex and type of diabetes.

It should be noted that there is some evidence from two studies that mean levels of serum cholesterol are higher in subjects with just impaired glucose tolerance than age-matched controls (Ostrander et al, 1980; Yano et al, 1982). This raises the possibility that abnormalities may even predate the onset of overt diabetes, and might date from adolescence or before (Tzagournis et al, 1968; Florey et al, 1976; Voors et al, 1981).

Studies are therefore mostly in agreement that hypercholesterolaemia and hypertriglyceridaemia are more prevalent in both Type 1 and 2 diabetic subjects, especially at diagnosis of diabetes. But the degree of diabetic control appears very important, as the best controlled diabetics may have lipid levels similar to non-diabetics (Wolff & Salt, 1958; Nikkila & Hormila 1978), whereas increasingly poor control may be associated with significant increases in serum lipids and lipoprotein levels (Sosenko et al, 1980). Diabetic treatment, particularly in Type 2 patients, may also have a profound effect. For example, higher levels of serum lipids are often associated with diabetic treatment of diet either alone or in combination with an oral hypoglycaemic agent when compared to those on insulin treatment (Lisch & Sailer, 1981). Likewise obesity appears to be an important determinant, with a trend for higher triglyceride levels to be observed in the more obese diabetic subjects (Braunsteiner et al, 1966; Nikkila & Hormila, 1978).

Recent attention has also been given to the diabetic with regard to ethnic differences in serum lipid levels which have been observed in the non-diabetic population. It appears that black males and females of West Indian origin have a strikingly lower prevalence of both hypercholesterolaemia and hypertriglyceridaemia compared to those of Asian or European extract (Pacy et al, 1985). These differences might, of course, partly contribute to the dissimilar patterns of cardiovascular disease seen in different ethnic groups (Cruickshank et al, 1980).

Lipoprotein Levels in Diabetes Mellitus

Several studies have reported that abnormal lipoprotein levels frequently accompany diabetes mellitus (Hayes, 1972; Garcia et al, 1974; Chase & Glasgow, 1976; Nikkila & Hormila, 1978; Mancini et al, 1980; Lisch & Sailer, 1981; Steiner, 1981). Abnormalities that may occur in poorly or newly diagnosed diabetes are shown in Table 4.2; these include increased VLDL and LDL levels in all types of diabetes as already mentioned, but with good diabetic control both these abnormalities may completely resolve (Nikkila & Hormila, 1978; Lisch & Sailer, 1981).

With regard to HDL levels, in general diabetic women have lower HDL-cholesterol levels than diabetic men when compared with non-diabetic controls (Gordon et al, 1977 a; Beach et al, 1979). However, there are differences between Type 1 and 2 diabetes: HDL levels are generally either normal or low in Type 2 diabetes (Lopes-Virella et al, 1977; Kennedy et al, 1978; Reckless et al, 1978; Taylor et al, 1981; Rendel et al, 1982): Studies on the subfractions have shown either an increase in the level of the HDL_3 subfraction (Durrington, 1982), or a reduction in HDL_2. Reduced lipoprotein lipase activity may give rise to low HDL levels and hypertriglyceridaemia in this type of diabetes. Other factors which may relate to lower HDL levels include poor diabetic control, increasing age, obesity, an inverse relationship to serum triglycerides, androgens, smoking and, although controversial, a high carbohydrate dietary intake (Ganda, 1980). Sulphonylurea therapy commonly instituted in diabetic subjects has also been implicated (Calvert et al, 1978), but more recently refuted (Taylor et al, 1982).

In contrast, HDL levels may be elevated or normal in Type I diabetic subjects (Garcia et al, 1974; Mattock et al, 1979; Lopes-Virella et al, 1983). The reason for an increase may be related to increased VLDL catabolism, which in turn produces the apoproteins and lipids forming an integral part of HDL.

With regard to HDL subfractions in insulin-dependent diabetics, data are conflicting but some studies have demonstrated a significant increase in HDL_3 in males but not in females (Mattock et al, 1980).

Other factors independent of diabetes which may elevate HDL levels in a particular patient include moderate alcohol intake (Hulley et al, 1979), exercise (Hartung et al, 1980), ethnic origin (Pacy et al, 1985) and oestrogens (Bradley et al, 1978). A reduction of HDL levels may also be caused by hypolipidaemic therapy, in particular probucol, and β-blocking drug therapy used in the treatment of hypertension (Dodson, 1982a).

Aetiology of Raised Triglyceride and VLDL Levels in Diabetes Mellitus

Insulin plays a crucial role in triglyceride and VLDL metabolism, particularly as the clearing enzyme lipoprotein lipase is dependent on insulin for its activity (Brunzell & Bierman, 1978). In insulin-deficiency states (as in Type 1 diabetes) lipoprotein lipase activity, estimated by post-heparin lipolytic activity, may be impaired with resultant hypertriglyceridaemia. If severe, this may result in the diabetic lipaemia that is particularly seen in poorly controlled or newly diagnosed diabetics (Bagdade et al, 1967). Restoration to normal circulating insulin levels promptly restores enzyme activity with a decrease in serum triglycerides (Kissebah et al, 1974).

The aetiology of hypertriglyceridaemia in Type 1 diabetics subsequently controlled and established on insulin is less clear but would appear to centre round the control and activity of lipoprotein lipase. Some studies have demonstrated no deficiency in lipoprotein lipase activity (Jones et al, 1966; Nikkila & Hormila, 1978), while others have suggested that there may be a relative deficiency of activity on prolonged stimulation with heparin infusion (Brunzell et al, 1973). It is therefore possible that subtle abnormalities of lipoprotein lipase activity may occur. It is probable that in most hypertriglyceridaemic insulin-dependent patients, the main defect is at the lipoprotein lipase level and hence there is a clearance defect.

A contributory factor in the mechanism of diabetic hypertriglyceridaemia may be increased free fatty acid turnover which is consistently found in uncontrolled diabetes (Lewis et al, 1972). As free fatty acids are the precursors of synthesis of triglyceride for incorporation into VLDL in the liver, it is not surprising that VLDL-triglyceride turnover may be increased in diabetics (Nikkila & Kekki, 1973). This may therefore give rise to increased endogenous triglyceride synthesis and release in the form of VLDL. This component of overproduction may therefore be an additional aetiology to that of the clearance defect described above. Some diabetics may also have underlying familial forms of hypertriglyceridaemia *per se* (Brunzell et al, 1979).

In contrast, in Type 2 diabetes, lipoprotein lipase activity is relatively intact (Nikkila et al, 1977) but overproduction of VLDL is the most likely cause of the hypertriglyceridaemia. The explanation for this may be that free fatty acids are released from adipose tissue in the presence of insulin resistance, and in the presence of increased circulating insulin levels an increase in hepatic synthesis of triglyceride will tend to occur, especially if the liver retains normal insulin sensitivity (Topping & Mayes, 1972; Kissebah et al, 1974). This will lead to enhanced VLDL formation and release. The situation may therefore be one of predominantly increased production of VLDL; however, it is also likely that a clearance defect is operative, as the rate of disappearance of intravenous Intralipid was reduced in a study of Type 2 diabetics, possibly due to low fatty acid incorporation into adipose tissue (Lewis et al, 1972).

The relative importance of increased se-cretion and/or impaired catabolism of circulating triglyceride in causing diabetic lipaemia has yet to be determined. However, it is probable that varying degrees of impairment of peripheral uptake of triglyceride interact with enhanced, normal or decreased secretion of VLDL to produce the wide range of lipid levels observed in untreated diabetes.

More recent research has identified structural abnormalities in the composition of VLDL in patients with hypertriglyceridaemia. These have consisted of altered ratios of the 'modulator' C-apolipoproteins found in VLDL. The obligate activator apo-C II has been shown to result in poor activation of lipoprotein lipase *in vitro* when present in very low or excess amounts in VLDL. Excess of Apo-C III 2 has also been demonstrated in diabetic subjects with severe hypertriglyceridaemia (Holdsworth et al, 1982). Catabolism of VLDL by lipoprotein lipase is impaired *in vitro* with this C-apoprotein abnormality and may therefore produce a clearance defect *in vivo*. Further research is needed in this area and it is possible that important abnormalities in the 'modulating' apoproteins may be found.

Aetiology of Raised Cholesterol and LDL Levels in Diabetes Mellitus

Cholesterol in the blood is mainly transported by LDL, and attention must therefore be focussed on LDL metabolism. The production of increased LDL levels is probably by three major mechanisms. The first is the suggestion of an absolute increase in LDL synthesis (Kissebah et al, 1976), which may be corrected by improved diabetic control (Bennion & Grundy, 1977). The second mechanism may be through the effect of insulin which actually may increase the number of LDL receptors at a cellular level (Chait et al, 1978). Therefore in insulin-deficient states a decrease in receptor numbers would be expected with consequent delay in LDL clearance.

The third mechanism is now well documented *in vitro* and involves non-enzymatic glycosylation of apoprotein B of LDL (Gonen et al, 1981; Kim & Kurup, 1982; Witzum et al, 1982). A 2- to 3-fold increase in the amount of glucose bound to lysine of apoprotein B has been demonstrated in the serum of diabetic subjects. This finding may be important, since it is known that chemical modification of lysine amino groups of the apoprotein may interfere with the specific LDL receptor binding and hence clearance of LDL (Gonen et al, 1981; Kim & Kurup, 1982; Witzum et al, 1982).

An interesting finding which may also be relevant is that there have been reports of a triglyceride-enriched LDL present in diabetics, regardless of type and treatment (Schonfeld et al, 1974; Mancini et al, 1980). The mechanism and pathophysiological significance of this abnormality remain unclear, but it may be a remnant particle accumulation which might in itself be atherogenic (e.g., like LDL).

Other factors, which might be contributory to hypercholesterolaemia in diabetics, include increased VLDL levels which contain a small amount of cholesterol, and a diet, high in total and saturated fat, that was previously employed in the treatment of diabetes.

Important Factors Influencing Lipid Levels

Diabetic control

A number of studies have suggested that good glycaemic control in diabetes may reverse a number of the lipid and lipoprotein abnormalities.

Hayes, in 1972, reanalysed lipid levels after short-term introduction of diabetic therapy. Good glycaemic control produced a reduction in the prevalence of hypercholesterolaemia from 52–12.5 per cent with a similar decrease in hypertriglyceridaemia (50–17.9 per cent). Longer term analysis still showed a reduction in the prevalence rates, but it was not as impressive. Other later short-term studies have confirmed these findings (Tamborlane, 1979; Dunn et al, 1981), and deterioration of glycaemic control has

also been shown to elevate lipid and lipoprotein levels (Sosenko et al, 1980; Lopes-Virella et al, 1981). Generally, the effect on triglyceride metabolism of excellent diabetic control is more profound than it is on cholesterol and LDL. Therefore, some authors have suggested that plasma lipid levels are a further test of diabetic control, and if abnormal levels are detected careful attention should be paid to improving blood glucose control.

Dietary effects

Dietary therapy has long been the cornerstone of diabetic management. The modern diabetic diet consists of high unrefined carbohydrate, and fibre, with a low fat content. Many studies have now shown that this sort of regimen improves total serum cholesterol and LDL levels in both insulin-dependent and non-insulin-dependent diabetics in the short and long term (Simpson et al, 1979 a, b; Dodson et al, 1981b). If more viscous fibres are used (e.g., guar gum preparations), more marked changes in serum cholesterol levels may be seen (Dodson et al, 1981b; Aro et al, 1981). Serum triglyceride levels are generally unaltered in both short- and long-term studies (Dodson et al, 1985), providing unrefined carbohydrate is used, as opposed to refined carbohydrate which has been shown to be hypertriglyceridaemic in some studies (Reaven, 1980). Recent studies of hyperlipidaemic diabetics treated with a high-fibre unrefined carbohydrate and low-fat content diet have demonstrated a significant reduction in both cholesterol and triglyceride levels on this type of diet (Pacy et al, 1984 a).

The situation with regard to HDL and its subfractions is unclear. Some short-term studies of the diabetic diet have shown either a reduction of HDL cholesterol (Rivellese et al, 1980; Simpson et al, 1981), no effect (Dodson et al, 1984) or significant elevations (Dodson et al, 1981 b). Data on HDL_2 are more scanty but it would appear that there may be an elevation of this subfraction in the longer term in diabetics on a dietary regimen similar to that currently recommended by the British Diabetic Association (Pacy et al, 1984 c).

The exact mechanisms of these effects are not entirely clear but are probably multifactorial and related to changes in improved diabetic control, dietary fat intake, and weight reduction. It would therefore appear that nutritional modifications in themselves have an important effect on serum lipids and lipoproteins. The current recommended diabetic dietary regimen appears to result in a reduction in lipid cardiovascular risk.

Alcohol intake, serum lipids and obesity

Alcohol may have several effects on serum lipids. These include enhancement of alimentary lipaemia if a meal is preceded by alcohol (Wilson et al, 1970 a), and chronic alcohol-related hyperlipidaemia in susceptible individuals. The main mechanism of these effects is probably increased incorporation of both dietary and endogenous fatty acids into VLDL by the small intestine (Lewis, 1976). Alcohol may also affect cholesterol metabolism by decreasing catabolism to bile acids (Lefevre et al, 1972).

The most frequent effect of excess alcohol intake on serum lipids is elevation of triglyceride levels. Severe lipaemia due to chronic alcohol abuse may result in recurrent attacks of pancreatitis and diabetes mellitus. In this situation there may be a familial hyperlipidaemia, the expression of which is heightened by alcohol ingestion or poor diabetic control.

Obesity is a common finding, particularly in Type 2 diabetes. Excess alcohol intake tends to contribute to obesity with increased VLDL production and an associated reduction of HDL levels.

Antihypertensive and other drug therapy

There has been recent concern with regard to the precipitation and aggravation of diabetes mellitus by thiazide diuretics (Murphy et al, 1982), and β-adrenoreceptor blocking agents and others used in the treatment of hypertension. These drugs may also adversely affect serum lipids and lipoproteins. A lowering of HDL-cholesterol, with elevation of serum cholesterol and triglyceride, has been well documented in non-diabetics (Goldman et al, 1980), but little studied in the diabetic. However, it would appear that serum triglyceride levels are significantly increased by thiazide diuretics in normolipaemic Type 2 diabetics, whereas in those formerly hyperlipidaemic there is only a minor increase (Gill et al, 1984; Pacy et al, 1984 a). β-blocking agents have been associated with similar effects (Dodson, 1982; Pacy et al, 1984 b), but HDL-cholesterol levels were not affected by either group of drugs in diabetic subjects (Dodson, 1982; Pacy et al, 1984 b).

Other therapeutic agents well known to adversely affect serum lipid levels include oestrogen-containing oral contraceptives, androgens, and moderate dosage of corticosteroid therapy.

Lipids Levels, Diabetes Mellitus and Atherosclerosis

Several studies have addressed possible relationships between macrovascular disease and serum lipids and lipoproteins but, whatever the contribution serum lipids make to macrovascular disease, many other interrelating factors have to be considered. Even so, using multivariate analysis to adjust for many of these, including cigarette smoking, sex, duration of diabetes, hypertension and obesity, the Framingham investigators concluded that all these are insufficient to account for the excess incidence of coronary heart disease, particularly in female diabetics (Garcia et al, 1974). However, as in the non-diabetic, data are available suggesting a link between serum lipids and, in particular, coronary heart disease.

A possible role for triglyceride in the pathogenesis of macrovascular disease of diabetes mellitus was postulated by Albrink in 1963 in a retrospective study of 139 patients (Albrink et al, 1963). He contrasted the lower plasma triglyceride levels and less evidence of atherosclerosis observed in the 1930s, with the higher levels of these features in the 1950s. Further evidence suggesting a positive link has been demonstrated in other cross-sectional studies (New et al, 1963; Ahuja et al, 1969; Santen et al, 1972; Albrink, 1974; Lamda et al, 1974; Reckless et al, 1978; Seviour et al, 1985). New found that fasting triglyceride levels were significantly higher in diabetics aged between 31–50 years with complications compared to those without, although no such relationship was observed in diabetics over 50 years of age (New et al, 1963). No association was found with cholesterol levels, but a distinction was made between macrovascular and microvascular complications in this study. Similar findings were recorded by Santen, who compared lipid levels in 52 diabetics with macrovascular disease, and a well age- and sex-matched normotensive control population (Santen et al, 1972). The mean fasting triglyceride and cholesterol levels in the diabetic macrovascular disease group were significantly higher than controls in the 30–59 age-group. In those aged 60–69 years similar trends were observed only for fasting triglyceride. The effect of obesity was considered but, although mean levels of triglyceride were increased by 28 per cent in obese subjects, the levels were still increased in lean diabetics with macrovascular disease compared to lean controls.

Albrink demonstrated a similar association in a subsequent study, with 82 per cent of diabetics greater than 50 years of age with clinically apparent atherosclerosis having triglyceride levels greater than 1.7 mmol/l compared to 50 per cent of those without atherosclerosis (Albrink, 1974).

In addition, several studies in diabetics have suggested that raised serum cholesterol levels are also associated with the presence of macrovascular disease. Lamda found that 68.2 per cent of diabetics had cholesterol levels greater than 6.5 mmol/l and, of the 23 diabetics with cholesterol levels above 7.75 mmol/l, 87 per cent had cardiovascular complications (Lamda et al, 1974).

Reckless reported a large series of 154 diabetics who were examined for the presence of macrovascular complications with relation to actual lipoprotein levels (Reckless et al, 1978). Clinical evidence of vascular disease was found in 38.3 per cent of patients and 30 per cent were hyperlipidaemic. Vascular disease was more common in those with higher concentrations of cholesterol, triglycerides, LDL and VLDL, and was less prevalent in those with higher HDL levels. In insulin-dependent patients and all male patients, cholesterol and LDL-cholesterol were positively associated with vascular disease but there was no inverse relationship with HDL. In the non-insulin-dependent diabetics and in all females, a strong inverse relationship was noted with HDL cholesterol. A weak positive association was only demonstrated with serum triglyceride, VLDL-triglyceride and LDL in females.

A more recent study in a small number of patients has emphasised these sex differences (Seviour et al, 1985). In 16 female Type 2 diabetic patients with clinically overt macrovascular disease, significantly higher serum triglyceride and lower total HDL-cholesterol levels were shown compared to those without macrovascular disease but who were well matched for age, duration of diabetes, weight and glycaemic control. Interestingly, HDL_2 subfraction levels were also studied with mean levels 79 per cent lower in those with macrovascular disease.

Although these cross-sectional studies suggest a similar positive relationship as in the non-diabetic between coronary heart disease and increasing serum cholesterol, triglyceride, VLDL and LDL levels, and possibly a negative association with HDL, confirmation of their contribution should be sought from prospective studies.

The Framingham Study, in 1974, reported a 16-year follow-up of diabetic patients but did not include measurement of HDL or LDL cholesterol. The subsequent Framingham Study in 1977 reported a shorter term follow-up and included serum lipids and lipoproteins in a multivariate analysis in a total cohort of 4939 subjects (Garcia et al, 1974). However, only 10.4 per cent of these were diabetic. A separate multivariate analysis of diabetics was not reported but, using standardised logistic regression coefficients for incidence of coronary heart disease, strong relationships were demonstrated in the whole group, as shown in Table 4.3. LDL-cholesterol levels were positively associated with coronary heart disease in both women and men, although this effect was stronger in men. Both sexes also demonstrated a strong negative relationship with HDL-cholesterol. However, serum triglyceride levels did not prove to be a significant factor for coronary heart disease in this multivariate analysis and this is probably because of the correction made for the inverse relationship between triglycerides and HDL. Thus in the Framingham Study, triglycerides do not appear to be an independent risk factor. This has also been supported by observations in Japanese and Hawaiian men (Chung et al, 1969), and is consistent with the low rate of macrovascular disease found in Pima Indians (Ingelfinger et al, 1976) and Bantu diabetics (Shapiro et al, 1973), in both of whom hypertriglyceridaemia is extremely common.

Prospective studies have also been performed in subjects with impaired glucose intolerance. In both the Whitehall and Hawaiian Studies (Fuller et al, 1980; Yano et al, 1982), increasing serum cholesterol levels carried a higher coronary disease mortality but multivariate analysis did not demonstrate serum cholesterol as an independent risk factor in either report.

It would therefore appear that, as in the non-diabetic, consistent evidence points to serum cholesterol and LDL-cholesterol as positive risk factors for coronary heart disease in the diabetic. HDL-cholesterol may also be a predictor with an inverse relationship, particularly in female diabetic subjects. Therefore, part of the explanation for diabetes mellitus conferring an increased incidence of vascular complications may be the adverse effects of diabetes on serum lipid and lipoprotein levels.

These conclusions are probably most valid for the female Type 2 diabetic subject, in whom it is interesting to speculate that serum lipid levels may have been towards the upper end of the normal distribution even in adolescence. Thus, by the time of diagnosis of diabetes in middle age, these subjects may have already had 30 years or more of exposure to these atherogenic factors (Jarrett, 1984).

Future clinical research will no doubt give us further insight into the role of lipid abnormalities in the development of macrovascular disease in the diabetic. Biochemical aspects which may also be important include further elucidation of the metabolism of HDL and its subfractions, the apoprotein B composition and its effect on LDL metabolism, and the interrelationships of serum lipids with other factors, for example, platelet function.

Diagnosis and Management of Hyperlipidaemia in Diabetic Subjects

Like moderate hyperglycaemia, significantly elevated lipid levels are often not associated with clinical features so patients need regular screening for hyperlipidaemia. The initial test of a random serum cholesterol and triglyceride estimation is sufficient. A random, as opposed to a fasting, sample has advantages as this can be performed in the routine diabetic clinic and in particular does not require a separate visit with alterations in timing of hypoglycaemic drug therapy.

Table 4.3 Multivariate analysis of serum lipid and lipoprotein levels, for the incidence of coronary heart disease in the Framingham Study, 1977

	Men		*Women*	
HDL-cholesterol	−0.61	$P<0.001$	−0.65	$P<0.001$
LDL-cholesterol	0.332	$P<0.01$	0.26	$P<0.05$
Triglyceride	−0.092	N.S.	−0.106	N.S.

N.S. Not significant.
Figures are standardised logistic regression coefficients from a cohort of 4939 subjects of whom 515 were diabetic.
Figure adapted from that of Gordon et al (1977a).
LDL, low density lipoprotein; HDL, high density lipoprotein (subfractions 2 and 3).

A random cholesterol estimation of greater than approximately 6.5 mmol/l in a diabetic patient aged less than 60 years should be repeated after a 12-hour overnight fast (and taken before morning hypoglycaemic therapy) on two further occasions to establish the diagnosis of hyperlipidaemia. The level of fasting cholesterol at which the diagnosis of hypercholesterolaemia is made will vary from clinic to clinic. In our clinic we have chosen >6.5 mmol/l in the under sixties for both sexes. We do not see the need for the level to be higher in diabetics than in non-diabetics. Above this level the rate of coronary heart disease increases steeply in non-diabetic prospective studies (Kannel et al, 1971; Goldbourt et al, 1985). Hypertriglyceridaemia is more difficult to define (Hulley et al, 1980), but it is our practice to institute active treatment of fasting serum triglyceride levels consistently 5 mmol/l or above in diabetic subjects when we are confident it is not secondary hypertriglyceridaemia.

When hyperlipidaemia is identified in a diabetic subject, attention must be focussed on diabetic control, obesity, diet, alcohol intake and drugs such as thiazides or β-blocking agents. The achievement of good glycaemic control, with $HbA_1 \leqslant 10$ per cent at a satisfactory body weight, is an essential first step in the management of diabetic hyperlipidaemia.

A common factor to improving diabetic control and weight loss is modification of dietary intake. The general dietary recommendations for diabetics of a diet high in fibre and unrefined carbohydrate, combined with a reduced fat content, appears to lower serum lipids as well as improving diabetic control in hyperlipidaemic diabetic subjects, and should therefore be advised (Pacy et al, 1984 a,c). Total energy content should be adjusted to obtain weight loss in obese subjects. Attention should be directed towards the type of fat consumed. Saturated table and cooking fats should be replaced with those of a polyunsaturated nature, a manoeuvre which has been shown to lower serum cholesterol levels (Keys et al, 1965).

Predisposing factors must be searched for and treated. For example, thyroid and renal disease, alcohol abuse and chronic pancreatitis may be identified. Attention should be focussed on concomitant drug therapy, for example, thiazide diuretics, which may be important aetiological factors.

It must be remembered that hyperlipidaemia in a well-controlled diabetic may also represent a primary familial disorder, and it is often difficult to differentiate between this and diabetes complicated by hypertriglyceridaemia. A careful family history and investigation of first-degree relatives may be helpful.

If hyperlipidaemia persists despite simple measures then drug therapy may be instituted. Combined hypercholesterolaemia and hypertriglyceridaemia is the common form requiring treatment. The agent of choice is one of the more recent clofibrate analogues (e.g., bezafibrate), which lowers both cholesterol and triglyceride levels by reducing cholesterol and triglyceride synthesis. This agent may also improve blood glucose control (Wahl et al, 1980).

If hypercholesterolaemia is a persisting problem then the anion-exchange resins, cholestyramine or colestipol, may be effective in lowering serum cholesterol by increasing the excretion of bile salts. When inadequate response occurs or there is difficulty in compliance owing to the need to ingest a large bulk of exchange resins, a further agent may be required (e.g., bezafibrate).

Severe lipaemia is rarely found but requires more urgent treatment. Cessation of alcohol abuse with which this condition is often associated may dramatically reduce the lipaemia, but other methods can be employed. These include continuous insulin infusion or plasma exchange. Severe lipaemia in an undiagnosed diabetic will usually resolve with the institution of insulin therapy and effective diabetic control.

However, it must be emphasised that generally hyperlipidaemia combined with diabetes mellitus can be adequately treated with attention to dietary measures, promoting weight loss and improving glycaemic control.

References

Ahuja, M.M.S., Kumar, V. and Gossain, V.V. (1969). Interrelationship of vascular disease and blood lipids in young Indian diabetics. *Diabetes* **18**, 670–674.

Albrink, M.J. (1974). Dietary and drug treatment of hyperlipidaemia in diabetics. *Diabetes* **23**, 913–918.

Albrink, M.J., Lavietes, P.H. and Mann, E.B. (1963). Vascular disease and serum lipids in diabetes mellitus: observations over 30 years (1931–1961). *Ann. Intern. Med.* **68**, 305–323.

Aro, A., Vusitupa, M., Vontilainen, E. et al (1981). Improved diabetic control and hypocholesterolaemic effect induced by long-term dietary supplementation with guar gum in type 2 diabetes. *Diabetologia* **21**, 29–33.

Bagdade, J.D., Porte, D. and Bierman, E.L. (1967). Diabetic lipaemia. A form of acquired fat-induced lipaemia. *N. Engl. J. Med.* **276**, 427–433.

Beach, K.W., Brunzell, J.D., Conquest, L.L. et al (1979). The correlation of arteriosclerosis obliterans with lipoproteins in insulin-dependent and non-insulin-dependent diabetes. *Diabetes* **28**, 836–840.

Bennion, L.J. and Grundy, S.M. (1977). Effects of diabetes mellitus on cholesterol metabolism in man. *N. Engl. J. Med.* **296**, 1365–1371.

Bradley, D.D., Wingers, J., Petitti, D.B. et al (1978). Serum high-density lipoprotein cholesterol in women using oral contraceptives, estrogens and progestins. *N. Engl. J. Med.* **299**, 17–20.

Braunsteiner, M., Sailer, S. and Sandhofer, F. (1966). Plasmalipide bei patienten mit diabetes mellitus. *Klin. Wochenschr.* **44**, 116–119.

Brunzell, J.D. and Bierman, E.L. (1978). Pathophysiology of lipoprotein transport. *Metabolism* **27**, 1109–1127.

Brunzell, J.D., Hazzard, W.R. and Motulsky, A.G. (1975). Evidence of diabetes mellitus and genetic forms of hypertriglyceridaemia as independent entities. *Metabolism* **24**, 1115–1121.

Brunzell, J.D., Porte, D. and Bierman, E.L. (1973). Evidence for a common, saturable, triglyceride removal mechanism for chylomicrons and very low density lipoproteins in man. *J. Clin. Invest* **52**, 1578–1585.

Brunzell, J.D., Porte, D. and Bierman, E.L. (1979). Abnormal lipoprotein lipase-mediated plasma triglyceride removal in untreated diabetes mellitus associated with hypertriglyceridaemia. *Metabolism* **28**, 901–907.

Calvert, G.D., Graham, J.J., Mannik, T. et al (1978). Effects of therapy on plasma-high-density-lipoprotein-cholesterol concentration in diabetes mellitus. *Lancet* **ii**, 66–68.

Castelli, W.P., Doyle, J.P., Gordon, T. et al (1977). HDL cholesterol levels and other lipids in coronary heart disease. The co-operative lipoprotein phenotyping study. *Circulation* **55**, 767–772.

Chait, A., Bierman, E.L. and Albers, J.J. (1978). Regulatory role of insulin in the degradation of low density lipoproteins by cultured human skin fibroblasts. *Biochim. Biophys. Acta* **529**, 292–299.

Chase, H.P. and Glasgow, A.M. (1976). Juvenile diabetes mellitus and serum lipids and lipoprotein levels. *Am. J. Dis. Child.* **130**, 1113–1117.

Chung, C.S., Bassett, D.R., Moellering, R.C. et al (1969). Risk factors for coronary heart disease in Hawaiian and Japanese males in Hawaii. *J. Med. Genet.* **6**, 59–66.

Committee of Principal Investigators (1978). WHO Clofibrate Trial: A cooperative trial in the primary prevention of ischaemic heart disease using clofibrate. *Br. Heart J.* **40**, 1069–1118.

Crall, F.V. and Roberts, W.C. (1978). The extramural and intramural coronary arteries in juvenile diabetes mellitus. Analysis of nine necropsy patients aged 19 to 38 years with onset of diabetes before age 15 years. *Am. J. Med.* **64**, 221–230.

Cruickshank, J.K., Beevers, D.G., Osbourne, V.L. et al (1980). Heart attack, stroke, diabetes and hypertension in West Indians, Asians and Whites in Birmingham, England. *Br. Med. J.* **281**, 1108.

Dayton, S., Pearce, M.L., Hashimoto, S. et al (1969). A controlled clinical trial of a diet high in unsaturated fat in preventing complications of atherosclerosis. *Circulation* **40**, Suppl. 2, 1–63.

Dodson, P.M. (1982a). Lipids and antihypertensive drug therapy. *Br. J. Clin. Pract.* **20**, Suppl., 17–20.

Dodson, P.M., Galton, D.J., Hamilton, A.M. et al (1982b). Retinal vein occlusion and the prevalence of lipoprotein abnormalities. *Br. J. Ophthalmol.* **66**, 161–164.

Dodson, P.M., Galton, D.J. and Winder, A.F. (1981a). Retinal vascular abnormalities in the hyperlipidaemias. *Trans. Ophthalmol. Soc. UK* **101**, 17–21.

Dodson, P.M., Pacy, P.J., Bal, P. et al (1984). A controlled trial of a high fibre, low fat and low sodium, diet for mild hypertension in Type 2 (non-insulin-dependent) diabetic patients. *Diabetologia* **27**, 522–526.

Dodson, P.M., Pacy, P.J. and Cox, E.V. (1985). Long term follow-up of the treatment of essential hypertension with a high fibre, low fat and low sodium dietary regimen. *Hum. Nutr. Clin. Nutr.* **39C**, 213–220.

Dodson, P.M., Stocks, J., Holdsworth, G. et al (1981b). High fibre and low-fat diets in diabetes mellitus. *Br. J. Nutr.* **46**, 289–294.

Dunn, F.L., Pietri, A. and Raskin, P. (1981). Plasma lipid and lipoprotein levels with continuous subcutaneous insulin infusion in type 1 diabetes mellitus. *Ann. Intern. Med.* **95**, 426–431.

Durrington, P.N. (1982). Serum high density lipoprotein cholesterol subfractions in type I (insulin-dependent) diabetes mellitus. *Clin. Chim. Acta* **120**, 21–28.

Florey, C. du V., Uppal S. and Lowy, C. (1976). Relation between blood pressure, weight, and plasma sugar and serum insulin levels in school children aged 9–12 years in Westland, Holland. *Br. Med. J.* **1**, 1368–1371.

Fuller, J.H., Shipley, M.J., Rose, G. et al (1980). Coronary heart disease risk and impaired glucose tolerance. The Whitehall Study. *Lancet* **i**, 1373–1376.

Galton, D.J., Stocks, J. and Dodson, P.M. (1982). Lipoproteins: their role in enzyme regulation. *Clin. Biochem. Rev.* **3** 377–405.

Ganda, O.P. (1980). Pathogenesis of macrovascular disease in the human diabetic. *Diabetes* **29**, 931–942.

Garcia, M.J., McNamara, P.M., Gordon, T. et al (1974). Morbidity and mortality in diabetics in the Framingham Population: sixteen-year follow-up *Diabetes* **23**, 105–111.

Gill, J.S., Al-Hussary, N., Atkins, T.W. et al (1984). Possible role for insulin receptors in the mechanism of thiazide induced glucose intolerance. *J. Hypertension* **2**, Suppl. 3, 573–576.

Glueck, C.J. (1977). Classification and diagnosis of hyperlipoproteinaemia. In Rifkind, B.M. and Levy, R.I. (eds), *Hyperlipidaemia, Diagnosis and Therapy*, New York, Brune & Stratton, pp. 17–39.

Goldbourt, U., Holtzman, E. and Neufeld, H.N. (1985). Total and high density lipoprotein cholesterol in the serum and risk of mortality: evidence of a threshold effect. *Br. Med. J.* **290**, 1239–1243.

Goldman, A.I., Steele, B.W., Schnaper, H.W. et al (1980). Serum lipoprotein levels during chlorthalidone therapy. *JAMA* **244**, 1691–1695.

Goldstein, J.L. and Brown, M.S. (1974). Binding and degradation of low density lipoproteins by cultured human fibroblasts. Comparison of cells from a normal subject and from a patient with homozygous familial hypercholesterolaemia. *J. Biol. Chem.* **249**, 5153–5162.

Goldstein, J.L. and Brown, M.S. (1977). The low-density lipoprotein pathway and its relation to atherosclerosis. *Ann. Rev. Biochem.* **46**, 897–930.

Gonen, B., Baenziger, J., Schonfield, G. et al (1981). Non-enzymatic glycosylation of low density lipoproteins *in vitro*. Effects on cell-interactive properties. *Diabetes* **30**, 875–878.

Gordon, T., Castelli, W.P., Hjortland, M.C. et al (1977a). Diabetes, blood lipids, and the role of obesity in coronary heart disease risk for women. *Ann. Intern. Med.* **87**, 393–397.

Gordon, T., Castelli, W.P., Hjortland, M.C. et al (1977b). High density lipoprotein as a protective factor against coronary heart disease. The Framingham Study. *Am. J. Med.* **62**, 707–714.

Gordon, V., Innerarity, T.L. and Mahley, R.W. (1983). Formation of cholesterol- and apoprotein E-enriched high density lipoprotein *in vitro*. *J. Biol. Chem.* **258**, 6202–6212.

Gordon, T., Kannel, W.B., Castelli, W.B. et al (1981). Lipoproteins, cardiovascular disease and death. The Framingham Study. *Arch. Intern. Med.* **141**, 1128–1131.

Hartung, G.H., Foreyt, J.P., Mitchell, R.E. et al (1980). Relation of diet to high-density-lipoprotein cholesterol in middle-aged marathon-runners, joggers and inactive men. *N. Engl. J. Med.* **302**, 357–361.

Hayes, T.M. (1972). Plasma lipoproteins in adult diseases. *Clin. Endocrinol.* **1**, 247–251.

Haylick, L. (1976). The cell biology of human ageing. *N. Engl. J. Med.* **295**, 1302–1308.

Holdsworth, G., Stocks, J., Dodson, P.M. et al (1982). An abnormal triglyceride-rich lipoprotein containing excess sialylated apolipoprotein C-III. *J. Clin. Invest.* **69**, 932–939.

Hulley, S., Ashamn, P., Kuller, L. et al (1979). HDL-cholesterol levels in the multiple risk factor intervention trial (MRFIT). *Lipids* **14**, 119–125.

Hulley, S.B., Rosenman, R.H., Bawol, R.D. et al (1980). Epidemiology as a guide to clinical decisions. The association between triglyceride and coronary heart disease. *N. Eng. J. Med.* **302**, 1383–1389.

Ingelfinger, J.A., Bennett, P.H., Liebow, I.M. et al (1976). Coronary heart disease in the Pima Indians. *Diabetes* **25**, 561–565.

Jackson, R.L., Morrisett, J.D. and Gotto, A.M. (1976). Lipoprotein structure and metabolism. *Physiol. Rev.* **56**, 259–316.

Jarrett, R.J. (1984). Type 2 (non-insulin-dependent) diabetes mellitus and coronary heart disease—chicken, egg or neither? *Diabetologia* **26**, 99–102.

Jones, D.P., Plotkin, G.R. and Arky, R.A. (1966). Lipoprotein lipase activity in patients with diabetes mellitus, with and without hyperlipemia. *Diabetes* **15**, 565–570.

Kannel, W.B., Castelli, W.P. and Gordon, T. (1979). Cholesterol in the prediction of atherosclerotic disease. *Ann. Intern. Med.* **90**, 85–91.

Kannel, W.B., Castelli, W.P., Gordon, T. et al (1971). Serum cholesterol, lipoproteins and the risk of coronary heart disease. The Framingham Study. *Ann. Intern. Med.* **74**, 1–12.

Kaufman, R.L., Assal, J.P., Soeldner, J.S. et al (1975). Plasma lipid levels in diabetic children. Effects of diet restricted in cholesterol and saturated fats.

Diabetes **24**, 672–679.

Kennedy, A.L., Lappin, T.R.J., Lavery, T.D. et al (1978). Relation of high density lipoprotein cholesterol concentration to type of diabetes and its control. *Br. Med. J.* **2**, 1191–1194.

Keys, A. (1970). Coronary heart disease in seven countries. AMA Monograph No. 29, Suppl. 1. *Circulation* **41**, 1–195.

Keys, A., Anderson, J.T. and Grande, F. (1965). Serum cholesterol response to changes in diet. The effect of cholesterol in the diet. *Metabolism* **14**, 759–763.

Kim, H.J. and Kurup, J.V. (1982). Non-enzymatic glycosylation of human plasma low density lipoprotein. Evidence for *in vitro* and *in vivo* glycosylation. *Metabolism* **31**, 348–353.

Kissebah, A.H., Adams, P.W. and Wynn, V. (1974). Interrelationship between insulin secretion and plasma free fatty acid and triglyceride kinetics in maturity onset diabetes and the effect of phenethyltrignanide (phenformin). *Diabetologia* **10**, 119–130.

Kissebah, A.H., Alfarsi, S., Adams, P.W. et al (1976). The metabolic fate of plasma lipoproteins in normal subjects and in patients with insulin resistance and endogenous hypertriglyceridaemia. *Diabetologia* **12**, 501–509.

Lamda, D.L., Singha, P. and Chandra, S. (1974). A study of diabetes in relation to blood groups and cholesterol levels. *Humangenetik* **23**, 51–58.

Lefevre, A.F., De Carli, L.M. and Lieber, C.S. (1972). Effect of ethanol on cholesterol and bile acid metabolism. *J. Lipid Res.* **13**, 48–55.

Lewis, B. (1976). *The Hyperlipidaemias*, Oxford, Blackwell Scientific Publications, pp. 303–311.

Lewis, B. (1983). The lipoproteins: predictors, protectors and pathogens. *Br. Med. J.* **287**, 1161–1164.

Lewis, B., Mancini, M., Mattock, M. et al (1972). Plasma triglyceride and fatty acid metabolism in diabetes mellitus. *Eur. J. Clin. Invest.* **2**, 445–453.

Lipid Research Clinics Program (1984). Primary prevention trial results. *JAMA* **251**, 365–374.

Lisch, H.J. and Sailer, S. (1981). Lipoprotein patterns in diet, sulphonylurea and insulin treated diabetics. *Diabetologia* **20**, 118–122.

Lopes-Virella, M.F. Wohltmann, H.J., Loadholt, C.B. et al (1981). Plasma lipids and lipoproteins in young insulin-independent diabetic patients: relationship with control. *Diabetologia* **21**, 216–223.

Lopes-Virella, M.F., Wohltmann, H.J., Mayfield, R.K. et al (1983). Effect of metabolic control on lipid, lipoprotein, and apolipoprotein levels in 55 insulin-dependent diabetic patients—a longtitudinal study. *Diabetes* **32**, 20–25.

Lopes-Virella, M.F.L., Stone, P.G. and Colwell, J.A. (1977). Serum high density lipoprotein in diabetic patients. *Diabetologia* **13**, 285–291.

Mancini, M., Rivellese, A., Rubba, P. et al (1980). Plasma lipoproteins in maturity onset diabetes. *Nutr. Metab.* **24**, Suppl. 1, 65–73.

Martin, G., Ogburn, C. and Sprague, C. (1975). Senescence and vascular disease. In: Cristafalo, V.J., Roberts, J. and Adelman, R.C. (eds), *Exploration in Ageing*, New York, Plenum Press, pp. 163–193.

Mattock, M.B., Fuller, J.H., Maude, P.S. et al (1979). Lipoproteins and plasma cholesterol esterification in normal and diabetic subjects. *Atherosclerosis* **34**, 437–439.

Mattock, M.B., Salter, A., Fuller, J.H. et al (1980). High density lipoprotein subfractions in insulin-dependent diabetics. *Diabetologia* **19**, 298.

Miller, N.E., Hammett, F., Saltissi, S. et al (1981). Relation of angiographically defined coronary artery disease to plasma lipoprotein subfractions and apolipoproteins. *Br. Med. J.* **282**, 1741–1744.

Miller, N.E., Thelle, D.S., Forde, O.H. et al (1977 a). High density lipoprotein and coronary heart disease: a prospective case-control study. *Lancet* **i**, 965–967.

Miller, N.E., Weinstein, D.B., Carew, T.E. et al (1977 b). Interaction between high density and low density lipoproteins during uptake and degradation by cultured human fibroblasts. *J. Clin. Invest.* **60**, 78–89.

Murphy, M.B., Lewis, P.J., Kohner, E. et al (1982). Glucose intolerance in hypertensive patients with diuretics, a fourteen-year follow-up. *Lancet* **ii**, 1293–1295.

New, M.I., Roberts, T.N., Bierman, E.L. et al (1963). The significance of blood lipid alterations in diabetes mellitus. *Diabetes* **12**, 208–212.

Nicoll, A., Duffield, R.G.M. and Lewis, B. (1981). Flux of lipoproteins into human arterial intima. *Atherosclerosis* **39**, 229–242.

Niehaus, C.E., Nicoll, A., Wootton, R. et al (1977). Influence of lipid concentrations and age on transfer of plasma lipoprotein into human arterial intima. *Lancet* **ii**, 469–471.

Nikkila, E.A. and Hormila, P. (1978). Serum lipids and lipoproteins in insulin treated diabetes. *Diabetes* **27**, 1078–1086.

Nikkila, E.A., Huttunen, J.K. and Ehnholm, C. (1977). Post heparin plasma lipoprotein lipase and hepatic lipase in diabetes mellitus. Relationship to plasma triglyceride metabolism. *Diabetes* **26**, 11–21.

Nikkila, E.A. and Kekki, M. (1973). Plasma triglyceride transport in diabetes mellitus. *Metabolism* **22**, 1–22.

Ostrander, L.D., Lamphiear, D.E., Block, W.D. et al (1980). Physiological variables and diabetic status: findings in Tecumseh, Mich. *Arch. Intern. Med.* **140**, 1215–1219.

Pacy, P.J., Dodson, P.M., Kubicki, A.J. et al (1984 a). Comparison of the hypotensive and metabolic effects of bendrofluazide therapy and a high fibre, low fat and low sodium diet in diabetic subjects with mild hypertension. *J. Hypertension* **2**, 215–220.

Pacy, P.J., Dodson, P.M., Kubicki, A.J. et al (1984 b). Comparison of the hypotensive and metabolic effects of metoprolol therapy with a high fibre, low sodium, low fat diet in hypertensive type 2 diabetic subjects. *Diab. Res.* **1**, 201–207.

Pacy, P.J., Dodson, P.M., Kubicki, A.J. et al (1984c). Effect of a high fibre, high carbohydrate dietary regimen on serrum lipids and lipoproteins in type 2 hypertensive diabetic patients. *Diab. Res.* **15**, 159–163.

Pacy, P.J., Dodson, P.M., Kubicki, A.J. et al (1985). Ethnic prevalence of hyperlipidaemia in hypertensive non-insulin-dependent (type 2) diabetic subjects. *Diab. Med.* **2**, 312A.

Patsch, J.R., Gotto, A.M., Olivercrona, T. et al (1978). Formation of high density lipoprotein 2-like particles during lipolysis of very low density lipoproteins *in vitro*. *Proc. Nat. Acad. Sci. USA* **75**, 4519–4523.

Reaven, G.M. (1980). How high the carbohydrate. *Diabetologia* **19**, 409–413.

Reckless, J.P.D., Betteridge, D.J., Wu P. et al (1978). High density and low density lipoproteins and prevalence of vascular disease in diabetes mellitus. *Br. Med. J.* **i**, 883–886.

Rendel, S.E.H., Elkeles, R.S. and Khan, S.R. (1982). High density lipoprotein and subfraction cholesterol: relation to type of treatment and control of diabetes. *Diabetologia* **22**, (abstract); 393.

Rivellese, A., Riccardi, G., Giacco, A. et al (1980). Effects of dietary fibre on glucose control and serum lipoproteins in diabetic patients. *Lancet* **ii**, 447–450.

Robertson, W.B. and Strong, J.P. (1968). Atherosclerosis in persons with hypertension and diabetes mellitus. *Lab. Invest.* **18**, 538–551.

Rosenman, R.H., Brand, R.J., Scholtz, R.I. et al (1976). Multivariate prediction of coronary heart disease during 8.5 year follow-up in the Western Collaborative Group Study. *Am. J. Cardiol.* **37**, 903–910.

Ross, R. and Glomset, J.A. (1976). The pathogenesis of atherosclerosis. *N. Engl. J. Med.* **295**, 369–77, 420–425.

Ross, R. and Marker, L. (1976.) Hyperlipidaemia and atherosclerosis. *Science* **193**, 1094–1100.

Rothblat, G.H. and Phillips, M.C. (1982). Mechanism of cholesterol efflux from cells. *J. Biol. Chem.* **66**, 375–402.

Santen, R.J., Willis, P.W. and Fajans, S.S. (1972). Atherosclerosis in diabetes mellitus. Correlations with serum lipid levels, adiposity and serum insulin levels. *Arch. Intern. Med.* **130**, 833–843.

Schonfeld, G., Birge, C., Miller, J.P. et al (1974). Apolipoprotein B levels and altered lipoprotein composition in diabetes. *Diabetes* **23**, 827–834.

Seviour, P.W., Teal, T.K., Richmond, W. et al (1985). Low HDL cholesterol and apoprotein A.I. in non-insulin-dependent diabetic females with macrovascular disease. *Clin. Sci.* **68**, Suppl. 11, p17.

Shapiro, D.J., Truswell, A.S. and Jackson, W.P.U. (1973). Comparison of serum cholesterol and triglyceride concentrations in white and Bantu diabetics. *S. Afr. Med. J.* **47**, 1445–1450.

Shattil, S.L., Anayo-Galindo, R., Bennett, J. et al (1975). Platelet hypersensitivity induced by cholesterol incorporation. *J. Clin. Invest.* **55**, 636–644.

Simpson, R.W., Mann, J.I., Eaton, J. et al (1979 b). Improved glucose control in maturity-onset diabetes treated with high-carbohydrate, modified-fat diet. *Br. Med. J.* **1**, 1753–1756.

Simpson, R.W., Mann, J.I., Eaton, J. et al (1979 a). High carbohydrate diets and insulin-dependent diabetics. *Br. Med. J.* **2**, 523–525.

Simpson, H.C.R, Simpson, R.W., Lousley, S. et al (1981). A high carbohydrate leguminous fibre diet improves all aspects of diabetic control. *Lancet* **i**, 1–5.

Small, D.M. (1977). Cellular mechanisms for lipid deposition in atherosclerosis. *N. Engl. J. Med.* **297**, 873–877.

Sosenko, J.M., Breslow, J.L., Miettinen, O.S. et al (1980). Hyperglycaemia and plasma lipid levels. A prospective study of young insulin-dependent diabetic patients. *N. Engl. J. Med.* **302**, 650–654.

Steiner, G. (1981). Diabetes and atherosclerosis: an overview. *Diabetes* **30**, Suppl. 2, 1–7.

Strandness, D.W., Priest, R.W. and Gibbons, G.E. (1964). Combined clinical and pathologic study of diabetic peripheral arterial disease. *Diabetes* **13**, 336–372.

Tall, A.R. (1979). Conversion of HDL_3 into an HDL_2-like particle *in vitro*. *Circulation* **60**, Suppl. 11, 72.

Tall, A.R. and Small, D.M. (1978). Plasma high-density lipoproteins. *New Engl. J. Med.* **299**, 1232–1236.

Tamborlane, W.V., Sherwin, R.S., Genel, M. et al (1979). Restoration of normal lipid and amino acid metabolism in diabetic patients treated with a portable insulin-infusion pump. *Lancet* **i**, 1258–1261.

Tan, M.H., Macintosh, W., Weldon, K.L. et al (1980). Serum high density lipoprotein cholesterol in patients with abnormal coronary arteries. *Atherosclerosis* **37**, 187–188.

Taylor, K.G., John, W.G., Matthews, K.A. et al (1982). A prospective study of the effect of 12 months treatment on serum lipids and apolipoproteins A-I and B in Type 2 (non-insulin-dependent) diabetes. *Diabetologia* **23**, 507–510.

Taylor, K.G., Wright, A.D., Carter, T.J.N. et al (1981). High density lipoprotein cholesterol and apolipoprotein A-I levels at diagnosis in patients with non-insulin dependent diabetes. *Diabetologia* **20**, 535–539.

Topping, D.L. and Mayes, P.A. (1972). The immediate effects of fructose and insulin on the metabolism of the perfused liver. Changes in lipoprotein secretion, fatty acid oxidation and esterification, lipogenesis and carbohydrate metabolism. *Biochem. J.* **126**, 295–311.

Tzagournis, M., Chiles, R., Ryan, J.M. et al (1968). Interrelationships of hyperinsulinism and hypertriglyceridaemia in young patients with coronary heart disease. *Circulation* **38**, 1156–1163.

Voors, A.W., Radhakrishnamurthy, B., Srinavasan, S.E. et al (1981). Plasma glucose level related to blood pressure in 272 children, ages 7–15 years, samples from a total biracial population. *Am. J. Epidemiol.* **113**, 347–356.

Wahl, P., Hasslacher, C.L., Lang, P.D. et al (1980). Lipid-lowering effect of bezafibrate in patients with diabetes mellitus and hyperlipidaemia. In Greten, H., Lang, P.D. and Schettler, G. (eds), *Lipoproteins and Coronary Heart Disease; New Aspects in the Diagnosis and Therapy of Disorders of Lipid Metabolism*, Baden-Baden, Gerhard Witzstrock, pp. 154–158.

Wilhelmsen, L., Wedel, H. and Tibblin, G. (1973). Multivariate analysis of risk factors for coronary heart disease. *Circulation* **48**, 950–958.

Wilson, D.E., Schreibman, P.H., Brewster, A.C. et al (1970 a). The enhancement of alimentary lipaemia by ethanol in man. *J. Lab. Clin. Med.* **75**, 264–74.

Wilson, D.E., Schreibman, P.H., Day, V.C. et al (1970 b). Hyperlipidaemia in an adult diabetic population. *J. Chronic Dis.* **23**, 501–506.

Witzum, J.L., Mahoney, E.M., Branks, M.J. et al (1982). Non-enzymatic glycosylation of low-density lipoprotein alters its biologic activity. *Diabetes* **31**, 283–291.

Wolff, O.H. and Salt, H.B. (1958). Serum lipids and blood sugar levels in controlled diabetics. *Lancet* **i**, 707–710.

Yano, K., Kagan, A., McGee, D. et al (1982). Glucose intolerance and nine-year mortality in Japanese men in Hawaii. *Am. J. Med.* **72**, 71–80.

Chapter Five

Platelets and Diabetes Mellitus

D.J. Betteridge

Dr John Betteridge obtained his BSc in biochemistry in 1969 and qualified MB BS from King's College Hospital Medical School in 1972. After Senior House Office appointments at the Royal Postgraduate Medical School and the Brompton Hospital, he moved to St Bartholomew's Hospital as Junior Registrar and subsequently as Research Fellow supported by an R.D. Lawrence Memorial Fellowship from the British Diabetic Association. He obtained his MD in 1979 following studies of lipid and lipoprotein metabolism in diabetic and hyperlipoproteinaemic subjects. From 1979 to 1981 he was Senior Registrar in Medicine at the Royal United Hospital in Bath and during that time carried out research into platelet function in diabetes and hyperlipoproteinaemic states. He was awarded his PhD in 1985. Dr Betteridge is currently Senior Lecturer in Medicine at University College, London, and Honorary Consultant Physician at University College Hospital. His main research interests are in the biochemistry of vascular disease in diabetes and hyperlipoproteinaemia.

Introduction

The already high incidence of vascular disease in non-diabetic western populations appears to be still higher in diabetic subjects and, although there have been suggestions of a specific diabetic large-vessel disease (Lundbaek, 1973), there is little evidence to suggest that atherosclerotic lesions in diabetics are distinct from those in non-diabetics (Strandness et al, 1964). However, atherosclerosis appears to be more extensive and to develop at an earlier age in diabetic patients (Robertson & Strong, 1968). These pathological findings are in agreement with clinical studies, the most convincing evidence coming from the prospective community study in Framingham. All major clinical manifestations of athero-

sclerosis were found to have an increased incidence in diabetics (Garcia et al, 1974).

Many factors may contribute to the increased incidence of large-vessel disease in diabetic patients, as in non-diabetic subjects; however, the increased incidence in diabetics has not been fully explained in terms of known risk factors (Jarrett et al, 1982). Therefore other metabolic abnormalities have been sought in diabetic subjects which might contribute to the increased vascular risk. In this chapter the possible role of enhanced platelet function in the development of diabetic vascular disease will be discussed because of the postulated role of platelets in early lesions of atheroma and their importance in the development of thrombus on pre-existing atheromatous plaques leading to final arterial occlusion. In addition, Colwell et al (1978) have postulated that abnormal platelet function secondary to the diabetic state may contribute to the development of the specific microvascular disease of diabetics which makes an important contribution to morbidity and mortality in the diabetic population, principally through retinopathy, nephropathy and neuropathy and possibly also a cardiopathy (Keen & Jarrett, 1982).

Structure and Physiology

Platelets which, like red blood cells, do not contain a nucleus, are the smallest of the formed elements of blood, circulating as biconcave discs approximately 2–3 μm in diameter. They are formed from megakaryocytes which, in the final process of maturation, become amoeboid in shape and their pseudopods penetrate the marrow sinusoids. These pseudopods fragment in the blood flow with the nucleus remaining in the bone marrow. The normal circulating count varies in man between 150 and 400 $\times$ 10^9/l and mean platelet survival is about 9.9 days. Platelets are removed from the circulation in the spleen and liver.

Platelets have a central role in normal haemostasis. Through their properties of adherence to vascular or foreign surfaces and their aggregation with other platelets they can initiate haemostasis. Platelets also participate in the fluid phase of coagulation through their active biochemical contents and by providing surfaces for reactions to take place. Platelets may also contribute to the development of atherosclerosis.

Structure

Platelet structure and its relationship to platelet function has been given tremendous impetus, through the application of electromicroscopy to the study of platelet anatomy and the development of techniques for isolation of physiologically active platelets and their preservation for ultrastructural study. The subject has been reviewed (White et al, 1981) and will be briefly described here (see Figure 5.1).

The peripheral zone comprises the platelet cell surface, the surface connected open canalicular system, the exterior coat or glycocalyx, the unit membrane and the submembrane region. The glycocalyx of platelets is thicker and more dense than surface coats of other blood cells and is rich in glycoproteins (Berndt & Phillips, 1981), which is not surprising bearing in mind the number of receptor functions and transport mechanisms active at the platelet surface. Using various surface-labelling probes many different glycoproteins have been identified on the platelet surface ($>$ 30) and some, notably Ib, IIb, III and IV, are present in high concentration and their functional roles are emerging.

The trilaminar unit membrane of the peripheral zone which provides the physiochemical separation between extracellular and intracellular constituents has important components including the sodium/potassium ATPase. The membrane lipids, important as sources of arachidonic acid for the cyclo-oxygenase reaction, are distributed asymmetrically with sphingomyelin and phosphatidyl choline on the outside and phosphatidyl inositol, phosphatidyl ethanolamine and phosphatidyl serine on the inner surface (Schick, 1979). The submembrane region contains a regular system of filamentous elements (White, 1969), which can be seen lateral to the circumferential band of microtubules in discoid platelets (Zucker-Franklin, 1970). These filaments, which are in close association with the cell membrane, may be concerned with the maintenance of platelet shape and in pseudopod formation in conjunction with actin-binding protein and α-actinin (Lucas et al, 1976; Schollmeyer et al, 1978).

The so-called sol–gel zone of platelets contains the important microtubules and microfilaments. Microtubules, of which tubulin is the major protein constituent, are located in a circumferential band in the equatorial plane just under the cell wall in discoid platelets, which suggests that they may be important in maintenance of the platelet cytoskeleton. In addition, microtubules may be involved in the internal align-

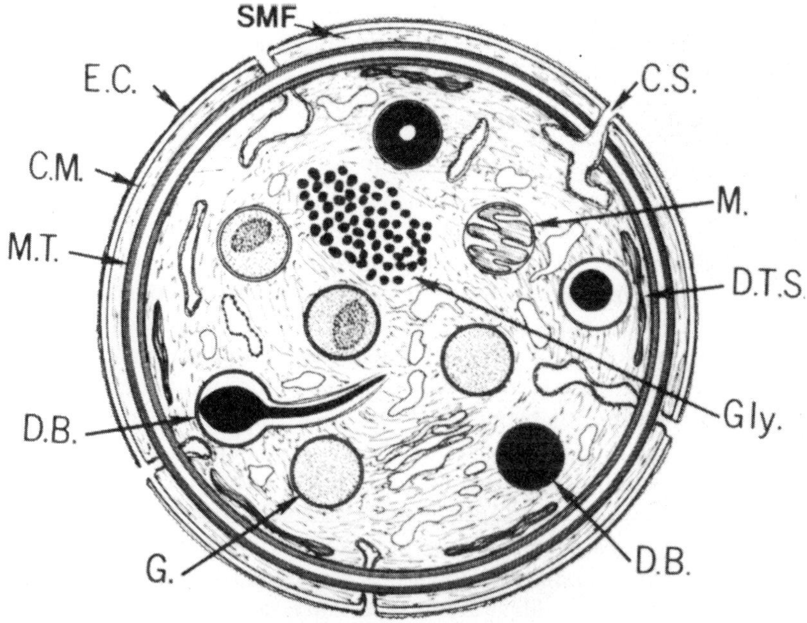

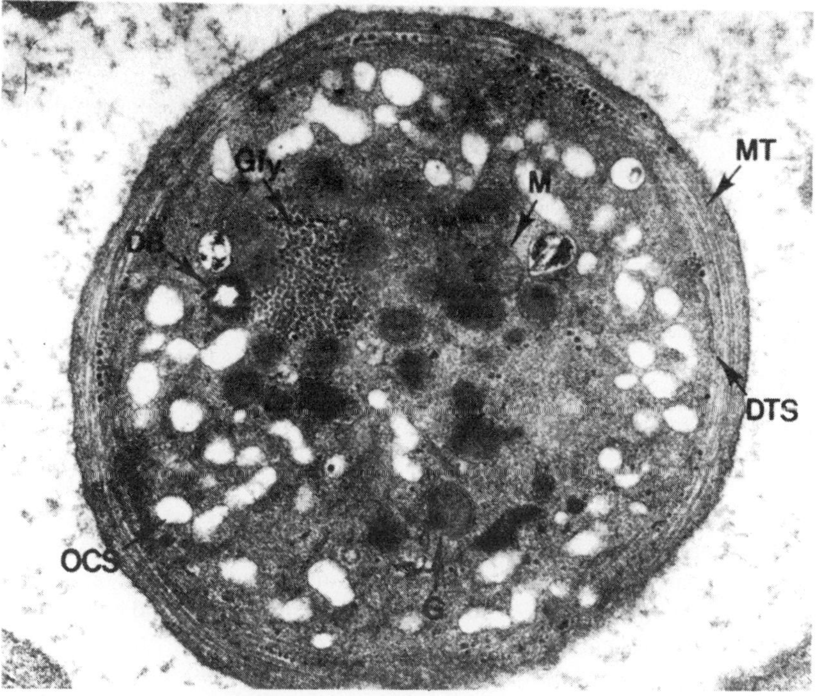

Figure 5.1 Platelet Ultrastructure. EC, exterior coat; CM, trilaminar unit membrane; SMF, sub-membrane filaments; CS, surface connected canalicular system; MT, microtubules; Gly, glyocogen; M, mitochondria; G, granules; DB, dense bodies; DTS, dense tubular system. White et al (1981). Reproduced by kind permission of Churchill Livingstone.

ment of platelet organelles before the release reaction and, furthermore, may help govern the degree of response to circulating agonists (White et al, 1981).

The second system of fibres in the sol–gel zone of platelets comprises the microfilaments (White, 1971). They resemble actin filaments found in other contractile cells such as muscle, and platelet actin has a 100-fold excess over platelet myosin (Pollard, 1975). The microfilament system provides the contractile capacity for the release reaction seen in activated platelets (Adelstein & Pollard, 1978). Cohen et al (1980) have postulated that the actin filaments are anchored to the platelet membrane by α-actin (glycoprotein III), a transmembrane protein. The actin filaments extend into the cytoplasm from this point and form long filaments orientated concentrically around the platelet granules. The myosin filaments would interdigitate between the actin filaments in opposite directions and help to push the platelet granules into the centre of the platelet for release into the surface-connected open canalicular system.

The platelet organelle zone is rich in several types of organelles. In addition to mitochondria, platelet cytoplasm contains numerous granules and dense bodies which have been distinguished by density, ultrastructural studies and biochemical content. The dense bodies (250–300 nm), so-called because of the electron-dense opaque internal content when visualized with the electron microscope, are the storage sites for 5-hydroxy-tryptamine, adenine nucleotides, calcium and pyrophosphate (Holmsen & Weiss, 1979). α-granules are the most numerous of platelet organelles and they have a variety of densities and staining characteristics. These granules (300–500 nm) store many proteins, some of which are specific to platelets such as platelet factor 4, β-thromboglobulin, low-affinity platelet factor 4 and platelet-derived growth factor. In addition α-granules contain proteins which are found in other cells and plasma such as fibrinogen, fibronectin, albumin and factor VIII-related antigen. It is probable that there are different types of α-granules with different granular contents which may be released in different situations (Kaplan, 1981). Platelets also possess a variety of lysosomal enzyme-storage organelles containing acid hydrolases including β-glucuronidase and β-galactosidase (Holmsen, 1975).

Platelets contain two important membrane systems, the surface-connected open canalicular system and the dense tubular system. The canalicular system consists of tortuous invaginations of the platelet wall running through the platelet cytoplasm and therefore greatly increasing the total surface area of platelet/plasma contact (Behnke, 1970). This system remains patent despite platelet contraction, adhesion and aggregation, and probably serves for the release of the contents of the platelet-storage granules to plasma (White, 1973). The dense tubular system which probably represents residual smooth endoplasmic reticulum is discrete from the open canalicular system (Behnke, 1970) but forms very close relationships with it in certain areas of the cytoplasm (White, 1972). An important physiologic role for the dense tubular system is calcium sequestration through the activity of the calcium/magnesium ATPase (Cutler et al, 1978).

Haemostasis

A series of complex reactions involving the vessel wall, plasma proteins and platelets occur to reduce the loss of blood following injury to the vasculature. Platelets contribute to these complex reactions in three main ways: they adhere to exposed collagen and form a physical plug to occlude the wound; they release active substances from their secretory granules which help to consolidate the initial platelet plug; they play an important role in interacting with the coagulation system and certain intrinsic coagulation reactions occur preferentially on the platelet surface. The process of platelet plug formation has been reviewed by Sixma & Wester (1977). Macroscopic observations of haemostatic plug formation have been made in animal models, particularly the hamster cheek pouch and the rabbit mesentery. Whereas transection of a capillary causes no bleeding, arterial transection results in vessel-wall contraction, retraction and brisk bleeding. Contraction is probably only important in the larger arteries and no contraction or retraction is seen when a vein is transected. Immediately following transection of the blood vessel there is accumulation of platelets on the exposed connective tissues at the edge of the wound. This is seen as a greyish-white accumulation of material which grows and obstructs blood flow. Eventually bleeding stops but may restart through channels in the platelet plug which are then occluded again. The haemostatic plug protrudes from the vessel and the blood behind the plug becomes stagnant.

Histological studies of platelet plug formation have been performed in animals and in biopsies of human skin followed bleeding time studies (Sixma & Wester, 1977; Wester et al, 1979). The earliest finding is the platelet adhesion to collagen fibres followed by aggregation and formation of a platelet plug. There is some fibrin formed at the edges of the wound and at the plug periphery but no fibrin is seen within the plug for about 15–30 minutes. In the first minute of the plug formation the platelets retain their granules and remain loosely packed. However, subsequently they become more closely packed and release their granules and the plug becomes a dense mass of interdigitated platelets. The major changes to the plugs in the hours following transection of the vessel are that lytic areas initially seen at the edges of the plug also develop in its centre and the degranulated platelets resemble empty vesicles. The pseudopodia disappear and the platelets appear round once more (Wester et al, 1979). In addition, there is increased fibrin formation with masses of fibrin between the platelets eventually forming a network of thick strands after 24 hours (Hovig et al, 1968). The platelet plays an important role in interacting with the coagulation system and certain intrinsic coagulation reactions occur preferentially on the platelet surface which appears to protect coagulation enzymes from inactivation by plasma proteinases and localises

fibrin formation within and around the platelet plug (Walsh, 1981). Fibrin deposition strengthens the platelet plug and the haemostatic barrier is complete. There is also infiltration of polymorphonuclear and mononuclear cells in the wound and sometimes in the plug itself and interestingly along the blood vessel near the wound (Wester et al, 1979).

As can be seen from the above description, the formation of the haemostatic plug or 'primary haemostasis' involves many properties of platelets including adhesion, aggregation, degranulation and release reaction, and these platelet properties will be briefly described.

Platelet adhesion

It is thought that the platelet is necessary for the maintenance of normal vascular integrity in that patients with thrombocytopaenia show a generalised haemorrhagic tendency and bruising when the platelet count falls below about $5 \times 10^9/l$, spontaneous bruising and more severe bleeding being possible as the platelet count falls below $20 \times 10^9/l$. In addition, haemorrhage can also occur due to qualitative platelet defects such as essential thrombocythaemia. The mechanism for the maintenance of this functional integrity is yet to be established, but presumably would involve platelet adhesion to the endothelium.

Platelets do not usually adhere to normal endothelium but the reasons why normal endothelium is inert with respect to stimulating platelet adhesion and aggregation is not fully understood (Shattil & Bennett, 1981). However, Moncada et al (1976a) demonstrated that endothelial cells were capable of producing a potent anti-platelet aggregatory agent and it was subsequently suggested that continuous production of this substance, now called prostacyclin, explained the apparent protection against adhesion and aggregation conferred by the normal endothelium (Moncada & Vane, 1979). Subsequent experimental work has cast doubt on this suggestion. For instance, in the rabbit, doses of aspirin sufficient to inhibit prostacyclin production do not lead to platelet adhesion to intact endothelium (Dejana et al, 1980). In addition, several studies have demonstrated that the amounts of prostacyclin normally found in the circulation are probably too low to have an appreciable effect on platelets (Steer et al, 1980; Haslam & McClenaghan, 1981; Greaves & Preston, 1982), and endothelial cells in culture produce little prostacyclin unless stimulated by thrombin for instance (Weksler et al, 1977).

Platelets will adhere to a variety of surfaces, both artificial and naturally occurring, the most important *in vivo* is the adhesion to collagen which occurs when the blood-vessel endothelium is damaged. This will be discussed later in this chapter.

Platelet aggregation

Platelet aggregation, or platelet–platelet stickiness, can be regarded as a special case of platelet adhesion and follows adhesion of platelets to injured surfaces. Normally, as has been described, aggregation is apparent in experimental wounds within seconds. Aggregation has been studied *in vitro* more than any other platelet activity because of the development of a simple photometric method for its measurement (Born, 1962). This is based on the observation that the optical density of stirred platelet-rich plasma (PRP) falls as aggregates develop and returns to normal as they disperse. Aggregation *in vitro*, which is an active process (Vargaftig et al, 1981), is dependent on pH, temperature, mechanical stirring, calcium-ion concentration, the concentration of platelets in the PRP and the time elapsed between the performance of the aggregation tests and the preparation of the PRP (Mills, 1981). Numerous natural and artificial substances are capable of causing platelet aggregation (Table 5.1), and depending on the nature of the aggregation agent and its concentration, aggregation may be reversible or irreversible and have one or two phases.

Adenosine diphosphate (ADP) was the first agent discovered that caused aggregation (Gaarder et al, 1961). ADP induces aggregation directly and leads to the platelet release reaction

Table 5.1 Platelet aggregation agents

Platelet aggregation agent	Reference
Adenosine 5′-diphosphate	Gaarder et al (1961)
Collagen	Zucker & Borelli (1962)
Thrombin	Grette (1962)
Adrenaline	Mitchell & Sharpe (1964)
5-Hydroxytryptamine	Mitchell & Sharpe (1964)
Immune complexes	Mueller-Eckhardt & Luscher (1968)
Platelet-activating factor	Benevist et al (1972)
Thromboxane A_2	Hamberg et al (1975)
Sodium arachidonate	Kinlough-Rathbone et al (1976)
Calcium ionophores	Massini & Luscher (1974)

(MacMillan, 1966). A single phase of aggregation followed by rapid disaggregation is seen with low concentrations of ADP. At threshold concentrations a second phase caused by ADP release from the platelets is seen and at high concentrations a single phase with irreversible aggregation is observed (Hardisty et al, 1970). Primary ADP-induced aggregation requires fibrinogen (Niewiarowski et al, 1971), which appears to be involved in early transitory interactions between platelets (Mustard et al, 1978). Other plasma protein co-factors, possibly adsorbed coagulation factors of the vitamin K-dependent group, may also be required (Miale & Kent, 1975). ADP may play a central role in the initiation of physiological platelet aggregation. This nucleotide is extruded from activated platelets and also may be derived from injured tissues and erythrocytes (Bergvist & Arfos, 1976).

At low concentrations of collagen, platelet aggregation is dependent on the release of arachidonic acid from platelet membrane phospholipid and the subsequent metabolism of arachidonic acid via the prostaglandin pathway (Packham, 1976). However, at higher concentrations collagen also causes release of ADP from platelet granules and this is independent of the prostaglandin pathway. For collagen to promote platelet aggregation it must possess its triple helical structure and must be present as fibrillar collagen (Zucker & Borelli, 1962).

Adrenaline induces a biphasic response when added to platelet-rich plasma (MacMillan, 1966). The first wave of aggregation induced by adrenaline is associated with uptake of calcium by platelets, and it has been suggested that a localised flux of calcium into the platelet plasma membrane enables the platelets to stick together (Gerrard et al, 1981). Unlike other aggregating agents (ADP, collagen and thrombin) adrenaline does not cause initial platelet shape change (seen as a transient increase in optical density of platelet-rich plasma). These other aggregating agents which cause shape change before platelet–platelet aggregation release calcium initially from an intracellular structure, probably the dense tubular system, so that there is an elevation in cytoplasmic calcium before plasma membrane calcium is altered (Gerrard et al, 1981).

The mechanisms by which platelet sticks to platelet during aggregation are not fully understood. However, extracellular calcium is necessary and there is considerable evidence, particularly from studies of thrombasthenic platelets, that the platelet surface glycoproteins IIb and III are involved (Nurden & Caen, 1974, 1975; Phillips & Agin, 1977). More recently, fibrinogen has been strongly implicated in platelet–platelet interactions. Platelets activated by thrombin were found to produce haemagglutinin activity with fixed bovine erythrocytes (Gartner et al, 1980), and subsequently the same group have shown that this agglutinin is bound to platelet membranes and appears in the incubation fluid following platelet activation by thrombin (Gartner et al, 1980). It is highly likely that this agglutinin is fibrinogen (Gartner et al, 1980; Berndt & Phillips, 1981). Indeed, the role of fibrinogen in platelet aggregation has been recognised for many years (Born & Cross, 1964; Brinkhaus et al, 1965). ADP-stimulated platelets exhibit increased fibrinogen binding and the features of the binding suggested a fibrinogen receptor on the platelet membrane which required extracellular calcium (Bennett & Vilaire, 1979; Peerschke et al, 1980).

Platelet-release reaction

The release of platelet-derived material and the profound biochemical and morphological changes that occur after platelet stimulation have been termed the platelet-release reaction (Grette, 1962). On stimulation, platelets release their dense bodies, α-granules and lysosome-like granules (see Table 5.2), but the integrity of the membrane structures, cytoplasm and mitochondria is preserved. Initial experiments were performed on porcine platelets stimulated by thrombin but subsequently many substances (secretagogues) have been found to provoke platelet aggregation: ADP, adrenaline and collagen as well as thrombin provoked release of 5-hydroxytryptamine and nucleotides from platelets (Mills et al, 1968). In addition, immune complexes (Humphrey & Jaques, 1955), arachidonic acid (Kaplan et al, 1979) and thromboxane A_2 (Hamberg et al, 1975) cause platelet release. More recently, the degranulating action of platelet-activating factor has been demonstrated (Chignard et al, 1979; McManus et al, 1979). Some secretagogues (e.g., ADP) stimulate the release of certain granules (dense bodies, some α-granules but not the lysosomal granules), whereas thrombin stimulates secretion of all types of granule including lysosomes (Holmsen, 1977). In addition to these 'physiological stimuli'

Table 5.2 Subcellular localisation of secreted platelet constituents.

α Granules	Dense granules	Lysosomes
Factor V	ATP	Acid hydrolases
Fibrinogen	ADP	
Albumin	Pyrophosphate	
Fibronectin	5-hydroxytryptamine	
Platelet factor 4		
Low-affinity platelet factor 4/β-thromboglobulin	Calcium	
Platelet-derived growth factors		

many 'non-physiological' stimuli stimulate platelet degranulation including calcium ionophores (Gerrard et al, 1974), lectins (Greenberg & Jamieson, 1974) and latex and viral particles (Holmsen, 1977). As reviewed by Skaer (1981) it is probable that there are many different types of granule. In addition, the response to various secretagogues in terms of which granules are released and to what extent varies. This suggests that platelets must possess very sophisticated intracellular control mechanisms.

Dense body contents are discharged through the platelet-surface membrane (Skaer, 1981), and this occurs from between 4 seconds and 3 minutes after addition of the secretagogue. Mobilisation of the internal calcium occurs after 0.75–1.8 seconds following the addition of thrombin (Feinstein, 1980). Therefore the release of intracellular membrane-bound calcium precedes the onset of the stimulus-induced degranulation. A further factor involved in the stimulus to degranulation may be the breakdown of phosphatidyl inositol wth the accumulation of diglyceride (Rittenhouse-Simmons, 1979) (1-stearoyl, 2-arachidonyl diglyceride). The diglyceride may be important in promoting membrane fusion of the dense body granule with the platelet-surface membrane and also as a substrate for the formation of prostaglandin endoperoxides and thromboxane A_2 which are powerful degranulation stimuli (Bell et al, 1979). In addition, the actual breakdown of the membrane polyphospoinositides by calcium-stimulated enzymes may promote degranulation as they have highly charged polar head groups which would tend to impede membrane fusion (Allan & Mitchell, 1979).

As has been seen, the platelet α-granules contain a large number of proteins and are very numerous in the platelet cytoplasm. For instance, α-granule fibrinogen forms approximately 10 per cent of the total platelet protein (Holmsen & Weiss, 1979). Not all α-granules may respond in the same way to secretory stimuli; for example, Zucker et al (1979), who found that over 80 per cent of platelet factor VIII-related antigen was present in the α-granules could only demonstrate the release of 30 per cent of this in response to stimulation with collagen. Similar findings have also been described for fibronectin (Ginsberg et al, 1979). Although there are several possible explanations for these findings as reviewed by Skaer (1981), it is possible that some α-granules may remain refractory to secretory stimuli.

The contents of the α-granules, unlike those of the dense bodies, are discharged into the open canalicular system. α-granule nucleoids have been demonstrated by electronmicroscopic studies in the canalicular system (White, 1974), and it is likely that normal secretion involves not only fusion of these granules with the canalicular system but also platelet contraction. The evidence for this is derived from the use of differing secretagogues (Gerrard et al, 1974).

Platelet prostaglandin metabolism

Over recent years there has been increasing interest in these widely distributed and biologically important compounds, and their importance in platelet biochemistry and platelet–vessel wall interactions has been emphasised.

The prostaglandins and thromboxanes are produced from certain 20-carbon atom polyunsaturated fatty acids with varying degrees of unsaturation. The most abundant of these acids in human tissue is arachidonic acid (Crawford, 1983). Most arachidonic acid is esterified in membrane phospholipid complexes, and in order to act as a substrate for the enzyme complex prostaglandin synthetase the free acid must be liberated by the action of phospholipase A_2. The activity of this membrane enzyme thus provides the first control step in the prostaglandin pathway by limiting the availability of arachidonic acid substrate (Figure 5.2).

Free arachidonic acid is then acted upon by the system of microsomal enzymes known as prostaglandin synthetase which is composed of cyclo-oxygenase and peroxidase activities. In the presence of molecular oxygen, the cyclo-oxygenase activity converts arachidonic acid to a 15-hydroperoxide endoperoxide known as prostaglandin G_2, which is then converted by the

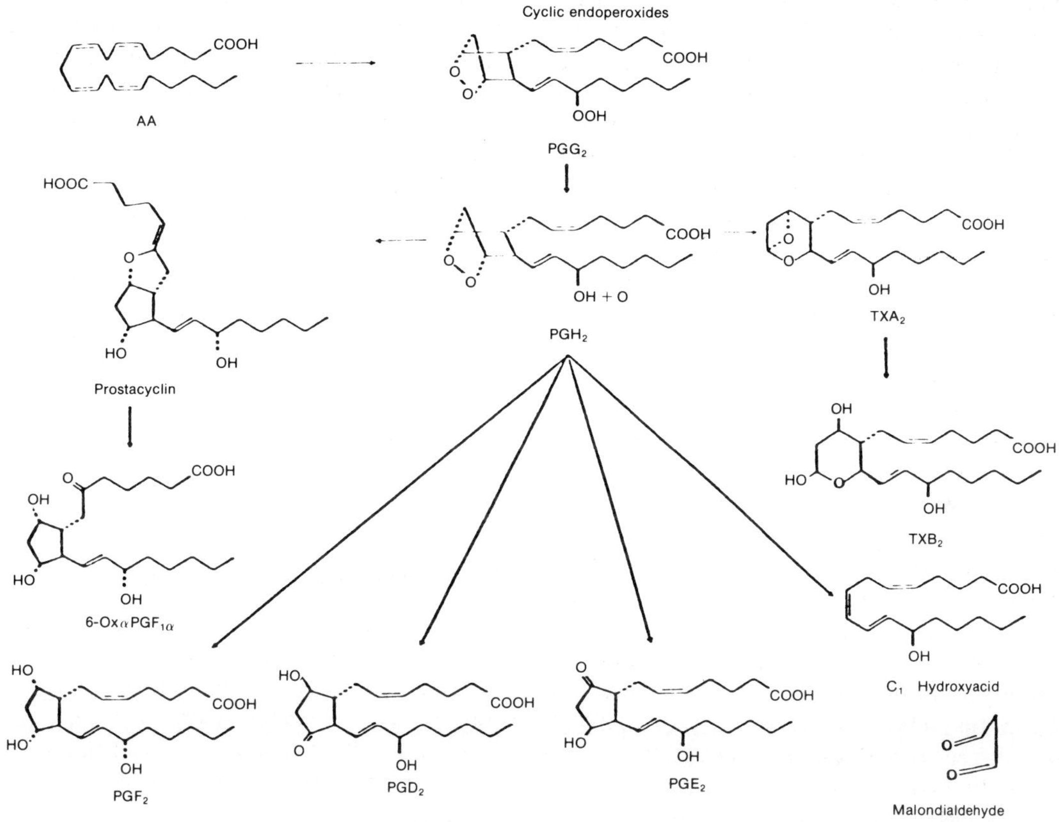

Figure 5.2 The prostaglandin pathway Arachidonic acid, AA; prostaglandin, PG; thromboxane, TX.

peroxidase activity to a 15-hydroxy endoperoxide known as prostaglandin H$_2$ (Lands, 1979) (see Figure 5.2). Prostaglandin H$_2$ is an unstable compound which has a half-life of approximately five minutes, and once formed is rapidly transformed either enzymically or non-enzymically to the classical prostaglandins, prostaglandin D$_2$, E$_2$ and F$_{2\alpha}$. Most tissues are capable of synthesizing these unstable endoperoxides and prostaglandins and it is products formed further along the prostaglandin pathway which determine the biological effects observed in different tissues. The synthesis of the prostaglandins E$_2$ and F$_{2\alpha}$ was demonstrated in platelets stimulated with thrombin by Smith and Willis (1971). These authors found that oral administration of aspirin was associated with

inhibition of platelet prostaglandin synthesis and suggested that this finding might explain the known effects of aspirin in inhibiting the platelet-release reaction and in prolonging the bleeding time (Quick, 1966). However, it was difficult to accept this concept as the prostaglandins measured were not proaggregatory. This was resolved a short time later when an unstable product of a short-term incubation of arachidonic acid with cyclo-oxygenase prepared from the vesicular gland of sheep was found to induce platelet aggregation (Willis & Kuhn, 1973). This product was subsequently found to be prostaglandin H$_2$ and the unstable endoperoxides prostaglandin G$_2$ and prostaglandin H$_2$ were found to be released during platelet aggregation (Hamberg et al, 1974). In addition, when these compounds were added to platelets they provoked aggregation (Hamberg & Samuelsson, 1974; Hamberg et al, 1974). Platelet aggregation induced by endoperoxides appeared to be greater than that which could be accounted for by the endoperoxides alone, and Hamberg et al (1975) were able to demonstrate that in platelets endoperoxides are further metabolised to a very unstable compound, thromboxane A_2. Thromboxane A_2 has a half-life of 30 seconds at body temperature and degrades spontaneously to the stable metabolite thromboxane B_2 (Hamberg et al, 1975). Subsequently, the microsomal fractions of human platelets have been shown to contain an enzyme which converts the endoperoxides, prostaglandin G_2 and H_2 to thromboxane A_2, and the enzyme has been designated thromboxane synthetase (Needleman et al, 1976). Thromboxane synthetase also catalyses the conversion of prostaglandin H_2 to a C-17 hydroxy acid known as 12-hydroxy-5.8.10-hepta-decatrienoic acid and malondialdehyde (Diczfalusy & Hammarström, 1977). However, prostaglandin H_2 conversion to these compounds may also occur non-enzymically (Van Dorp et al, 1978). It appears from experiments in which platelet-membrane fractions have been separated that thromboxane synthesis is associated with intracellular membranes known as dense tubular membranes (Carey et al, 1982).

Platelets can also metabolise arachidonic acid by a lipoxygenase enzyme system to yield a variety of hydroxy acids via their respective hydroperoxide intermediates (Hamberg & Samuelsson, 1974; Nugteren, 1975). The biological activity of these compounds remains to be determined. However, 12-L-hydroperoxy-5,8,10, 14-eicosatetraenoic acid may inhibit prostacyclin synthetase and cyclo-oxygenase (Siegel et al, 1979).

In 1976, a new relatively inactive arachidonic acid metabolite characterised as 6-oxo-prostaglandin $F_{1\alpha}$ was isolated from several tissues including guinea-pig lung (Dawson et al, 1976). In the same year, Moncada et al (1976a) reported the presence of an enzyme in aortic tissue which converted prostaglandin endoperoxides to a potent unstable inhibitor of platelet aggregation. This factor also relaxed arterial smooth muscle and was named prostaglandin X (Moncada et al, 1976 a). Prostaglandin X rapidly lost activity in neutral and acidic media with the formation of a relatively inert substance subsequently identified as 6-oxo-prostaglandin $F_{1\alpha}$, and prostaglandin X was identified as 9-deoxy-6, 9-epoxy-Δ^5-prostaglandin $F_{1\alpha}$ and renamed prostacyclin (Johnson et al, 1976). The microsomal enzyme converting prostaglandin H_2 to prostacyclin was named prostacyclin synthetase and prostacyclin was found to be the major product of arachidonic acid in the walls of arteries and veins in several animal species and man (Moncada & Vane, 1978). However, prostacyclin synthetase although present in many tissues is not present in platelets (Moncada & Vane, 1979).

Thromboxane A_2 is a more powerful proaggregatory substance in platelets than the endoperoxides, and it has been proposed that it is the arachidonic acid metabolite that mediates platelet aggregation and the release reaction (Hamberg et al, 1975). Whether platelet endoperoxides have a proaggregatory role in their own right or only when converted to thromboxane A_2 has been the subject of many studies (Bunting et al, 1983). However, from experiments using thromboxane synthetase inhibitors it appears that when platelets are activated and the prostaglandin cascade is triggered by release of endogenous arachidonic acid then the endoperoxides generated exert their proaggregatory effects by their conversion to the more potent compound thromboxane A_2. However, when the thromboxane generation is suppressed it is probable that endoperoxides can be proaggregatory themselves (Bunting et al, 1983).

It has been proposed that endoperoxides and thromboxane A_2 activate platelets by acting as calcium ionophores, hence mobilising intracellular free calcium (Gerrard et al, 1978). However, all prostaglandins that induce platelet aggregation cause a monophasic reversible 'primary' response at low concentrations and a monophasic irreversible 'secondary' response at high concentrations. In this way the activation of platelets by prostaglandins resembles that produced by ADP and adrenaline. This is unlike the activation induced by the powerful stimulus of calcium ionophores in that prostaglandins induce platelet dense body secretion and α-granule secretion but not secretion of lysosomal hydrolases (MacIntyre, 1979). For this reason and others (reviewed by MacIntyre, 1981), including studies with antagonists, desensitisation experiments and measurement of calcium ionophore activity, it is thought that platelet activation by prostaglandins and thromboxanes is receptor-mediated although a suitable radiolabelled ligand is not available for definitive demonstration (MacIntyre, 1981).

Defreyn et al (1981) have demonstrated a deficiency of thromboxane formation and platelet aggregation in platelets from a patient with a familial bleeding tendency, thus emphasizing the importance of thromboxane production in the physiology of platelet function.

Thromboxane A_2 is a powerful vasoactive compound, and the activity of the rabbit aorta-contracting substance released from sensitized guinea-pig lungs described by Piper and Vane (1969) is accounted for by this substance (Hamberg et al, 1975). Because of its highly unstable nature, various thromboxane A_2-generating systems have to be used in order to study its vasoactive properties. Using these techniques it has been shown that thromboxane A_2 is a potent contractor of isolated vessel segments from several species including coronary arteries from pig and cattle, human umbilical artery and rabbit aorta (Moncada & Vane, 1979). In addition, strips of bovine cerebral conductance arteries and human basilar arteries contract with thromboxane A_2 (Boullin et al, 1979; Ellis et al, 1979).

The effect of thromboxane A_2 on differing vascular preparations has also been studied *in vivo* using thromboxane synthesized *in vitro* by incubations of endoperoxide with platelet microsomes. Using this technique, Dusting et al (1978) were able to show short-term vasoconstriction in femoral and vascular beds of the dog following injection of the thromboxane close to the vessels.

Prostacyclin has powerful metabolic effects on blood platelets. It has the most potent effect of the naturally occurring prostaglandins in inhibiting platelet aggregation, being 30–40 times more potent than prostaglandin E_1 and 10 times more potent than prostaglandin D_2 *in vitro* (Gryglewski et al, 1976; Moncada et al, 1976a). Prostacyclin can also bring about disaggregation of platelet aggregates *in vitro* (Moncada et al, 1976 a; Ubatuba et al, 1979). In addition, using animal models, prostacyclin applied locally has been shown to inhibit thrombus formation in response to ADP in the hamster cheek pouch microcirculation (Higgs et al, 1977), and given systemically prostacyclin inhibited thrombus formation induced electrically in rabbit carotid artery (Ubatuba et al, 1979). Similar findings were observed with prostacyclin either applied locally or given systemically in the coronary artery of dog (Aiken et al, 1979).

When given systemically prostacyclin protected against sudden death (secondary to platelet aggregation) in the rabbit following intravenous injection of arachidonic acid (Bayer et al, 1979). Gryglewski et al (1978) incorporated collagen strips into extracorporeal circuits in animals and showed that prostacyclin brought about disaggregation of platelet aggregates formed on the collagen strips. Similarly, prostacyclin inhibited platelet aggregation on rabbit subendothelium but only prevented platelet adhesion at higher doses (Higgs et al, 1978). In man prostacyclin infusion inhibited platelet aggregation measured *ex vivo* at a threshold dosage of 2 ng/kg/min, and with increasing doses there was increased inhibition of ADP-induced aggregation (Fitzgerald et al, 1981).

Although platelets cannot synthesize prostacyclin they do possess the enzyme 9-hydroxy-prostaglandin dehydrogenase (Wong et al, 1980). This enzyme can transform 6-oxo-prostaglandin $F_{1\alpha}$, the stable hydrolysis product of prostacyclin, into 6-oxo-prostaglandin E_1 which does possess antiaggregatory effects (Quilley et al, 1980). However, the possible biological role of this metabolite in platelet function remains to be determined, as plasma levels of 6-oxo-prostaglandin E_1 (measured by gas chromatography, mass spectrometry techniques) did not increase following intravenous infusion of prostacyclin (Jackson et al, 1982).

The potent inhibitory action of prostacyclin on platelet aggregation correlates with its ability to stimulate the platelet adenylate cyclase system, thus increasing cyclic AMP levels within the cell (Tateson et al, 1977). Stimulation of adenylate cyclase follows binding of prostacyclin to a platelet membrane receptor which it shares with prostaglandin E_1 but is distinct from the prostaglandin D_2 receptor (Miller & Gorman, 1979). Shepherd et al (1983) have calculated that each human platelet has 4200 high-affinity binding sites for prostacyclin with a dissociation constant of 16 nmol. In keeping with its stronger anti-platelet aggregatory effects compared to prostaglandin E_1, prostacyclin stimulation of adenylate cyclase activity is more potent and more sustained (Gorman et al, 1977). By enhancing platelet cyclic AMP levels through its stimulation of adenylate cyclase, prostacyclin can reduce cytoplasmic calcium levels which determine platelet shape change, aggregation and the release reaction (Käser-Glanzmann et al, 1977). In addition, platelet phospholipase A_2 (Minkes et al, 1977) and cyclo-oxygenase (Malmsten et al, 1976) are inhibited by the elevated cyclic AMP levels.

Prostacyclin is the major product of arachidonic acid metabolism in blood vessels and the synthesis is highest in the intima (Moncada et al, 1977). Capillaries also generate prostacyclin (Goehlert et al, 1981) and studies with cultured cells have demonstrated that it is endothelial cells which are the main source (Weksler et al, 1977). Thus when endothelium was stripped from rabbit aorta *in vivo* prostacyclin production at the luminal surface of the vessel was virtually absent and recovery of prostacyclin production was slow over a period of 70 days coinciding with the appearance of neointimal cells (Eldor et al, 1981).

Prostacyclin in contrast to thromboxane A_2 produced relaxation in most arterial preparations tested *in vitro* and was a potent vasodilator when tested in isolated perfused heart preparations (reviewed by Moncada and Vane, 1979). In addition, Dusting et al (1979) demonstrated increased blood flow in the coronary arteries of the intact heart in open-chested dogs following application of prostacyclin. Prostacyclin is a potent vasodilator in the microcirculation as demonstrated using the hamster cheek pouch preparation by Higgs et al (1982) and in the cerebral microcirculation of the cat by Ellis et al (1979).

In intact experimental animals prostacyclin has a vasodepressor effect and this was observed to an equal degree when injected intravenously or intra-arterially (Armstrong et al, 1978). This work suggests that prostacyclin is not inactivated in the pulmonary circulation unlike other prostaglandins. However, the vascular activity of prostacyclin *in vivo* is very short-lived and is less than its chemical half-life at physiological temperature and pH (i.e., $<$ three minutes). This suggests that biological inactivation takes place very rapidly *in vivo* and that most metabolites of prostacyclin have little vasodepressor activity apart from 6-oxo-prostaglandin E_1 (reviewed by Whittle and Moncada, 1983).

Platelets, Thrombosis and Atherosclerosis

Thrombosis

Platelets are undoubtedly involved in the final occlusion of atheromatous arteries and form the major component (the 'white head' of aggregated platelets) of the occlusive thrombus (Davies & Thomas, 1981). This sudden and often catastrophic event is most likely precipitated by fissuring of an underlying atheromatous plaque, as detailed analysis of obstructed coronary arteries at postmortem invariably shows that the thrombus is found in association with haemorrhage into a plaque. (Chapman, 1965; Constantinides, 1966; Friedman, 1970). In addition to their apparent central role in the pathogenesis of the arterial thrombus, increasing interest has focussed on platelets and the coronary microcirculation with the finding of platelet aggregates in the coronary microcirculation in some cases of sudden cardiac death (Haerem, 1972; El-Maraghi & Genton, 1980). These findings have stimulated an increasing amount of research into the mechanisms involved yet the pathogenesis of thrombus formation remains to be clarified. Certainly platelets do not normally adhere to arterial endothelium if it is not damaged but the explanation for this antithrombotic property of intact endothelium remains obscure. Following the discovery of prostacyclin it was suggested that endothelial cell production of this very potent antiaggregatory substance might explain this important property (Moncada et al, 1977; Moncada & Vane, 1978). However, this suggestion has not been confirmed experimentally, as has been discussed previously. Platelets will rapidly adhere and aggregate if the endothelial barrier is breached, as has been shown in many studies in experimental animals (reviewed by Mustard et al, 1983), and platelets adherent to collagen release the contents of their α and dense granules. Fissuring of an atherosclerotic plaque would also expose collagen fibres, and the adhering platelets could release agents such as thromboxane A_2 and ADP, which would rapidly lead to adhesion and aggregation of more platelets and growth of the thrombus. In addition, prostacyclin generation is probably reduced in the region of the atherosclerotic plaque, possibly due to the high content of lipid peroxides in advanced atherosclerotic lesions (Glavind et al, 1952). It is known that fatty acid peroxides inhibit prostacyclin generation (Moncada et al, 1976 b; Salmon et al, 1978). Thus the production of prostacyclin by cultured smooth muscle cells obtained from plaques of the experimental atherosclerotic rabbit consistently produced less prostacyclin when compared to control cells (Larrue et al, 1980). Furthermore, prostacyclin production measured by bioassay and 6-oxo-prostaglandin $F_{1\alpha}$ concentrations was reduced in perfused heart preparations from atherosclerotic rabbits

(Dembinska-Kiec et al, 1977). Similarly, prostacyclin production in human atherosclerotic tissue appears to be reduced. Sinzinger et al (1979) demonstrated decreased prostacyclin generation from atherosclerotic tissue compared to normal arterial tissue and could find no difference between early and advanced lesions. D'Angelo et al (1978) found no prostacyclin generation in atheromatous plaques from three subjects. In addition to the probable decreased prostacyclin production in the region of the atheromatous plaque possibly due to inhibition of prostacyclin synthetase by lipid peroxides it is known that certain fatty acid hydroperoxides also induce platelet aggregation (Mickel & Horbar, 1974). Thus diminution of prostacyclin production and stimulation of platelet aggregation both mediated by lipid peroxides could contribute to thrombosis on atheromatous plaques.

Increased thromboxane A_2 production may also contribute to thrombogenesis in atherosclerotic vessels. Thus platelet thromboxane A_2 production (measured as the stable degradation form thromboxane B_2) is increased in patients with arterial or venous thrombosis (Lagarde & Dechavanne, 1977) and myocardial infarction (Szczeklik et al, 1978). Similarly, following acute ligation of the coronary artery in dogs, high levels of thromboxane B_2 were found to be associated with cardiac arrhythmias (Coker et al, 1981). In addition, thromboxane B_2 levels were found to be elevated in the peripheral blood of patients with Prinzmetal angina (Lewy et al, 1979; Robertson et al, 1981) and in coronary sinus blood of patients with unstable angina (Hirsh et al, 1981).

Although the above description of experimental findings would suggest that exposure of collagen and lipid peroxides due to rupture of the atheromatous plaque could be of importance in thrombogenesis, together with enhanced platelet thromboxane A_2 formation and diminished vessel wall prostacyclin formation, Born has questioned this series of events (Born, 1983). He has pointed out that platelet aggregates grow very rapidly and, although platelet adhesion to collagen is almost instantaneous, there is a lag period (several seconds) before aggregation proceeds (Wilner et al, 1969). In addition, mural platelet thrombi can occur during passage of anticoagulated blood through artificial extra-corporeal systems (Richardson et al, 1976), which suggests that under certain circumstances collagen or other vessel wall constituents are unnecessary for activation of platelets. Born has assembled evidence to suggest that the important trigger to thrombogenesis *in vivo* is ADP and that at sites of vascular injury enough ADP is released from damaged cells to initiate thrombogenesis (Born, 1983).

Whatever the physiological stimulus to plate-let aggregation and thrombus formation it appears that it is the fissuring of an athero-matous plague often with extrusion of plaque lipid contents which triggers thrombus formation (Bouch & Montgomery, 1970). The nature of this obviously very important event remains unclear. However, a possible explanation has been put forward by Brooks et al (1971), which proposes that softening of the atheromatous plaque may be due to the presence of unusual lipids (cholesteryl esters of hydroxyoctadecadienoic acid) found in high concentrations in ulcerated plaques (Harland et al, 1971) which are thought to produce smooth muscle cell necrosis at the base of the plaque.

Atherogenesis

As has been discussed above, platelets are a crucial factor in thrombogenesis associated with atheromatous arteries. However, over recent years the possible role of platelets in the early stages of the atheromatous process has been emphasised (Ross & Glomset, 1976). Of course the advanced atherosclerotic plaque is a very complex structure, but the early lesion is very much a process which involves the intima of the artery and is characterised by proliferation of smooth muscle cells which have migrated from the media of the artery (Woolf, 1983). The fact that this early lesion is intimal suggests a response to a factor or factors in the blood, and

the 'response to injury' hypothesis is central to current thinking on the atherosclerotic process. It was Virchow in the middle of the nineteenth century who first put forward the concept of arterial wall injury leading to the development of the atheromatous plaque. In the middle of the twentieth century Duguid (1946) emphasised the importance of arterial thrombi in the genesis of the plaque and pointed out that it was Rokitansky who first put forward the 'encrusta-tion hypothesis'. The role of platelets in the process (which has resulted from the work of several groups: (Chandler & Hand, 1961; Murphy et al, 1962; French, 1966; Ross et al, 1974) as put forward by Ross and Glomset (1976) is really a bringing together of the Virchow and Rokitansky hypotheses of more than a century ago in that platelets may themselves contribute to vessel injury, thrombosis and atherogenesis (Mustard et al, 1983).

The functions of the endothelial cells of the arterial intima have been reviewed by Majno and Joris (1978), who highlighted several important aspects of endothelial cell physiology. These included: a barrier function to the formed elements of blood and plasma macromolecules; resistance to platelet thrombi; active transport of substances from blood; synthesis of factors involved in vessel wall–blood interactions and vascular repair processes. Thus endothelial cells synthesise many elements of their underlying connective tissue including fibronectin, elastin, collagen, proteoglycans and microfibrils (Buonassisi, 1973; Howard et al, 1976; Jaffe et al, 1976; Bornstein & Sage, 1980) which controls vessel permeability as well as stimulating throm-bosis following loss or damage to endothelial cells (Smith et al, 1979). Exchange of macro-molecules across the endothelium involves active vesicle formation, and transendothelial channels and intercellular clefts (Simionescu et al, 1976; Chien, 1978). The resistance of intact endo-thelium to platelet aggregation does not solely depend on its ability to synthesize prostacyclin as has been discussed previously. Other factors which may be involved in this important property are: secretion of plasminogen activator

(Loskutoff & Edgington, 1977), a membrane-associated ADPase (Lieberman et al, 1977), the presence of heparin-like membrane proteoglycans (Thorgeirsson & Robertson, 1978); the ability to take up and degrade vasoactive amines (Johnson & Erdos, 1977) the uptake and clearance of circulating thrombin (Lollar & Owen, 1980) and surface charge (Sawyer & Srinivasan, 1973).

From the above description it can be seen that the endothelial cell has many important properties and endothelial damage is proposed as the initial event in the 'response to injury' hypothesis. In the postulated series of events breach of the endothelial barrier would expose sub-endothelial smooth muscle cells and connective tissue to plasma constituents including lipoproteins, platelets and macrophage-type mononuclear cells (Harker & Ross, 1979). Following endothelial injury, platelets would adhere to the injured site, form microthrombi and release their granular contents which include a potent α-granule-derived mitogen that stimulates migration and focal proliferation of intimal and medial smooth muscle cells (Ross & Vogel, 1978). Subsequently there would be synthesis of collagen, elastin and proteoglycans by smooth muscle cells, intracellular and extracellular lipid accumulation and thrombosis associated with the lesion. Support for this sequence of events has come from animal models of atherosclerosis and studies using cell-culture techniques, and as Born (1983) has pointed out caution is necessary in translating these findings to the human situation. However, there does seem to be considerable evidence linking platelets to the development of proliferative arterial intimal lesions following experimental removal of endothelium in animal experiments, either mechanically or chemically (reviewed by Mustard et al, 1983). In addition, the emerging information regarding the properties of the platelet-derived growth factor argues for an important role in the atherogenic process of this platelet α-granule constituent.

Platelet-derived growth factor has been highly purified and appears to consist of two polypeptide chains of molecular weight 14 000–17 000 covalently joined by disulphide bonds (reviewed by Bowen-Pope and Ross, 1984). Following its purification it has been possible to study the biological properties of platelet-derived growth factor. Important amongst these properties are its ability to: induce chemotaxis by vascular smooth muscle cells (Grotendorst et al, 1982); fibroblasts (Seppä et al, 1982) and monocytes (Deuel et al, 1982); increase rates of fluid phase pinocytosis (Davies & Ross, 1978) and protein synthesis (Owen et al, 1982); increase the number of LDL receptors (Chait et al, 1980) and somatomedin receptors (Clemmons et al, 1980) as well as stimulate proliferation of connective tissue cells. It remains to be seen whether cells can respond to platelet-derived growth factor *in vivo* and, at the moment, its role in atherogenesis remains speculative but attractive.

As has been discussed, the 'response to injury' hypothesis depends on initial endothelial injury and little is known about loss of endothelium *in vivo* either spontaneously or in response to risk factors for atherosclerosis. Although endothelial replication is increased in response to hypertension or hyperlipidaemia (Florentin et al, 1969; Schwartz et al, 1980), this does not necessarily imply that the arterial intima is denuded of endothelium. In addition, studies with the electronmicroscope have not shown significant areas of denuded intima in early hyperlipidaemia in animal models despite there being increased endothelial turnover (Taylor et al, 1978). These findings have led to the suggestion that altered endothelial function without endothelial loss may be important in permitting platelet thrombus formation. In this regard, Gryglewski et al (1978) showed that prostacyclin formation in segments of blood vessel from cholesterol-fed monkeys was reduced. These authors, on the basis of these experiments, suggested a primary role for prostacyclin deficiency in the development of atherosclerosis in these animals. However, this suggestion depends on the assumption that prostacyclin is continually produced by arterial wall to prevent platelet aggregation. This assumption is not tenable as it is now recognised that the unstimulated output of prostacyclin by blood vessels is low (reviewed by Dollery et al, 1983). However, factors that reduce the ability of the vascular endothelium to produce prostacyclin may impair the ability of the vessel to respond to vascular injury (Dollery et al, 1983).

Recent work (Faggiotto & Ross, 1984; Faggiotto et al, 1984) has cast more light on the 'response to injury' hypothesis in cholesterol-fed monkeys. These workers have emphasised that the initial lesion in this model of atherogenesis is the adherence to endothelium of monocytes which then appear to migrate into the subendothelium, accumulate lipid and become lipid-laden macrophages or foam cells. It was only after some months that endothelial denudation was observed with platelet mural thrombus attached to exposed lipid-containing macrophages. These authors postulate that in as yet an unexplained way it is the accumulation of these lipid-laden foam cells in the sub-endothelium that damage the endothelium, thus allowing the subsequent developments in the formation of the atheromatous plaque to proceed.

Platelet Function in Diabetes Mellitus

Introduction

Despite increasing numbers of research communications concerned with platelet function in the diabetic there remain many conflicting reports and unresolved questions. Many factors contribute to this unsatisfactory situation. For instance, there is no absolutely satisfactory test of platelet function. Many studies have been performed using *in vitro* tests and it is difficult to be certain of the relevance of these tests to platelet function *in vivo*. Platelets are studied in an artificial environment and the very process of preparing the platelet sample for study may affect their behaviour. However, there is no doubt that the development of the turbidometric method for the study of platelet aggregation *in vitro* (Born, 1962) gave tremendous impetus to the study of platelet function. In more recent

years, as understanding of platelet physiology has increased, newer tests have been applied to the study of platelets from diabetic subjects which may be more relevant to platelet function *in vivo*. It has become possible to measure plasma levels of β-thromboglobulin and platelet factor 4 which are specific platelet proteins (Niewiarowski, 1977; Moore et al, 1975). They are stored within platelet α-granules (Niewiarowski, 1977) and are released to the surrounding plasma during platelet aggregation induced by thrombin, collagen, ADP, adrenaline and various lectins (Holmsen et al, 1969, 1975). β-Thromboglobulin (MW 35 000) is the most abundant specific platelet protein and its platelet concentration is $30–10^4$ times higher than in other tissues (Ludlam, 1979). Since it is cleared from human plasma with a half-life of 100 minutes (Dawes et al, 1978) an elevated plasma β-thromboglobulin level may be a useful indicator of enhanced *in vivo* platelet activation and 'release reaction'. Platelet factor 4 has a very short half-life (Musial et al, 1980) compared to β-thromboglobulin, which therefore makes it less sensitive for the detection of the '*in vivo*' platelet-release reaction, but it is a useful measure of artefactual *in vitro* secretion during and after blood sampling (Kaplan & Owen, 1981).

In recent years the importance of the prostaglandin pathway in platelets in relation to platelet aggregation has become apparent and several studies have attempted to assess the activity of this pathway in platelets from diabetic subjects. In addition, prostaglandin metabolism may play a crucial role in the interaction between platelets and vascular endothelium and several studies have examined the effect of the diabetic state on prostacyclin synthesis and the balance between prostacyclin and thromboxane.

Further attempts to estimate platelet function *in vivo* have involved isotopic labelling of platelets and measurement of platelet survival and assessments of platelet aggregation in whole blood. However, all these tests have potential limitations and results must be interpreted with caution.

In addition to problems intrinsic to the

methodology of platelet function, problems also arise from the diabetic groups studied. Many of the early studies of platelet function in diabetic subjects failed to take into account other factors known to influence platelet function, particularly the presence or absence of diabetic vascular complications. This has led to difficulties in interpretation of the possible sequence of events in the development of enhanced platelet reactivity in diabetics. In other words, are observed platelet abnormalities related to the disturbed metabolic state of diabetes or are they secondary to the presence of vascular disease? More recent studies have attempted to overcome this problem by electively studying diabetics free from clinical evidence of vascular disease. However, it is difficult to be completely sure of the absence of vascular disease on clinical grounds alone and, for this reason, some groups have studied platelet function in diabetic children and adolescents in whom vascular disease would be unlikely.

Platelet-adhesion studies

Early studies of platelet function in diabetes used *in vitro* tests of platelet adhesion. A variety of techniques were used involving glass beads or fibres in a column. Anticoagulated blood or platelet-rich plasma was passed through the column at a fixed flow rate and platelet counts were performed before and after exposure to these foreign surfaces — the difference being the number of platelets adhering. In general these techniques are tricky and difficult to reproduce and conflicting results were reported. Whereas increased platelet adhesion was reported in diabetics with evidence of microvascular and macrovascular disease (Mayne et al, 1970), no increase in adhesion was found in diabetics with retinopathy (Heath et al, 1971). However, the majority of studies did show increased adhesiveness in diabetic subjects with (Valdorf-Hansen, 1967; Badawi et al, 1970; Hellem, 1971) and without (Shaw et al, 1967; Hellem, 1971) vascular disease.

Platelet aggregation

Turbidometric studies

For *in vitro* aggregation studies citrated blood is carefully centrifuged to produce platelet-rich plasma. Aliquots of platelet-rich plasma are then placed in an aggregometer and stirred at 37°C. Various agonists, for example, ADP, collagen, adrenaline and thrombin, are then added to the platelet-rich plasma to induce aggregation which is measured as a change in optical density.

Studies of *in vitro* aggregation in diabetics date from the late sixties and early seventies. These early studies were performed in diabetics with and without clinical evidence of vascular disease. However, as Colwell et al have pointed out (Colwell et al, 1983) if enhanced platelet aggregation were to contribute to the pathogenesis of diabetic vascular disease then evidence of it should be present before the development of vascular disease. Later studies have taken care to define the diabetic population studied in terms of the presence or absence of complications. Increased platelet aggregation has been reported in patients with neuropathy (O'Malley et al, 1975) retinopathy (Heath et al, 1971; Bensoussan et al, 1975) and coronary artery disease (Szirtes, 1970). However, conflicting findings have appeared. For instance, in a study of 25 retinopathy patients — the marker most commonly used for microvascular disease — platelets exhibited enhanced platelet aggregation to the agonists adrenaline and arachidonic acid but not to ADP (Creter et al, 1978). On the other hand, platelet sensitivity to ADP was exaggerated in retinopathy patients studied by Khosla et al and was significantly greater than that in diabetics without retinopathy (Khosla et al, 1979).

The majority of reports of platelet-aggregation studies in diabetics without clinical evidence of vascular complications have found increased aggregation to various agonists, particularly ADP and collagen (Sagel et al, 1975; Halushka et al, 1977; Stuart et al, 1979; Halushka et al, 1981 a; Silberbauer et al, 1981; Janka et al, 1983). However, the occasional study has failed to demonstrate increased platelet aggregation in diabetics free of vascular disease (Petersen & Gormsen, 1978; Corbella et al, 1979) and certainly it would appear from the studies as a whole that platelet aggregation is more enhanced in diabetics with complications.

Platelet aggregation in whole blood

Recently a new method of measuring platelet aggregation has been described (Cardinal & Flower, 1980) which enables platelet aggregation in response to various agonists to be studied in whole blood. When two electrodes are suspended in whole blood, a monolayer of platelets will form and the conductance between the electrodes is constant. However, further platelets aggregate to the platelet monolayer when an aggregation agent is added and an accretion of platelets occurs between the two electrodes. This resulting increase in impedance between the electrodes may be observed on a pen recorder. This may be a more physiological approach to the study of platelet aggregation as platelets are studied immediately after blood sampling in the presence of red cells, white cells and the heavier platelets that are removed by the centrifugation step in techniques using platelet-rich plasma. These cells may be important modulators of platelet function *in vivo* through their ability to take up adenine nucleotides and synthesize and release regulatory prostaglandins (Roos & Pfleger, 1972; Blackwell et al, 1978). In addition, important regulators of platelet function, such as prostacyclin and cyclic AMP, may have been degraded to inactive products during the time taken to prepare platelet-rich plasma.

This technique has been applied to the study of platelet function in diabetic subjects (Jones et al, 1985). In response to the agonist arachidonic acid (1 mM) which acts via the prostaglandin pathway, and collagen (1 μg/ml) which acts partly directly by adhesion and also via prostaglandin synthesis, whole blood samples from the diabetic subjects showed increased platelet aggregation. No significant differences were seen with the higher dose of collagen (5 μg/ml), probably because the impedance aggregometer is more sensitive to smaller platelet aggregates than to the larger aggregates which would have been induced by the high-dose collagen (Ingerman-Wojenski et al, 1982). The diabetics chosen for this study were free of clinical evidence of vascular disease, which suggests that the platelet abnormalities in this diabetic group were due to the diabetic state (Jones et al, 1985).

Spontaneous platelet aggregation

Several studies have attempted to assess whether there is evidence of increased circulating platelet aggregates in diabetic subjects. The platelet aggregate ratio as described by Wu and Hoak (1974) depends on the ratio of the platelet count performed on platelet-rich plasma derived from blood mixed with formalin to that in platelet-rich plasma prepared without formalin. Formalin fixes platelet aggregates which would be removed during the centrifugation to produce platelet-rich plasma. Therefore the platelet-aggregate ratio would be low in the presence of circulating platelet aggregates.

It is important to remember that other factors may affect the platelet-aggregate ratio such as the rate at which blood is drawn through the sampling needle (Rohrer et al, 1978). However, Davis et al demonstrated that a group of 15 insulin-dependent diabetics without clinical evidence of complications had a significantly reduced platelet aggregate ratio of 0.75 ± 0.6 ($\pm$ s.d.) compared to age- and sex-matched control subjects with a ratio of 0.91 ± 0.11 (Davis et al, 1982). No difference in the platelet-aggregate ratio was found between a group of 15 diabetics diagnosed after the age of 30 years (six treated with insulin), some of whom had vascular complications compared to age- and sex-matched controls. No details were given of the glycaemic control or other metabolic parameters of the two groups of diabetics studied (Davis et al, 1982), and it is difficult to account for these findings. Dettori et al (1983) assessed the platelet-aggregate ratio in 92 'adult onset' diabetics and compared the results to 50 control subjects of a similar age. No differences were observed in the diabetic group as a whole compared to controls. However, when the patients were divided into those with good control ($HbA_{1c} < 9$ per cent) and bad control ($HbA_{1c} > 9$ per cent) it was found that the group with poor control had a significantly reduced platelet-aggregate ratio. Along with this there was a highly significant inverse relationship between platelet-aggregate ratio and HbA_{1c}. No such correlation was seen with various parameters of lipid metabolism (Dettori et al, 1983). In a further study of the platelet-aggregate ratio in diabetic subjects, Preston et al found a significant reduction in the diabetic group and this was due mainly to those diabetics with evidence of microvascular complications (Preston et al, 1978).

The above studies have attempted to assess the presence of circulating platelet aggregates. Other studies have measured 'spontaneous' platelet aggregation in platelet-rich plasma and whole blood *in vitro* using a variety of techniques but mostly involving agitation by stirring. The platelet aggregates formed in this way are fixed with formol. It is difficult to assess the significance of 'spontaneous' platelet aggregation, that is platelet aggregation induced by stirring alone without the addition of an aggregatory agent. However, the phenomenon is unusual in healthy individuals and it is conceivable that circulation stresses may have similar effects on platelets *in vivo*. Studies of this kind have demonstrated increased spontaneous *in vitro* platelet aggregation in insulin-dependent diabetic subjects free from vascular disease (Krzywanek & Breddin, 1981; Paulsen et al, 1981; Silberbauer et al, 1981).

Platelet-specific proteins

Initial reports of β-thromboglobulin levels in diabetic subjects were conflicting. Whereas in one study no significant increase in β-thromboglobulin was found (Campbell et al, 1977), other studies revealed higher levels of β-thromboglobulin in diabetic patients (Burrows et al, 1978; Preston et al, 1978). It has been suggested that the different findings in these studies were due to the different techniques applied to the collection of blood samples. In the study of Campbell et al blood samples were collected into plastic tubes containing PGE_1 in addition to EDTA and theophylline (Campbell et al, 1977). In the other studies PGE_1 was not present in the sample tubes (Burrows et al, 1978). However, it is now generally accepted that β-thromboglobulin levels are elevated in diabetics (Davis et al, 1979) and further evidence came from a large study of β-thromboglobulin and platelet factor 4 in diabetics compared to age- and sex-matched controls (Betteridge et al, 1981). It is known that there is a significant increase in the level of β-thromboglobulin with age (Ludlam et al, 1975; Zahavi et al, 1980) and a sex difference in old healthy subjects (Zahavi et al, 1980). Both β-thromboglobulin and platelet factor 4 levels were significantly elevated in diabetics compared to age- and sex-matched controls (Betteridge et al, 1981). Levels of β-thromboglobulin and platelet factor 4 were highly significantly correlated both in control subjects and diabetic patients, confirming that these two proteins are released from the same platelet pool and presumably at the same rate. A significant positive correlation was found between β-thromboglobulin and malondialdehyde formation in washed platelets stimulated by arachidonic acid. Malondialdehyde is a stable end-product of the prostaglandin pathway in platelets. The significant positive correlation of β-thromboglobulin to platelet malondialdehyde formation suggests that the enhanced platelet-release reaction may be in part linked to increased platelet prostaglandin synthesis in diabetic subjects (Betteridge et al, 1981), possibly leading to generation of unstable endoperoxides and thromboxanes which are powerful inducers of platelet aggregation and release reaction (Hamberg et al, 1975).

β-Thromboglobulin levels have been shown to be elevated in various types of vascular disease. Ludlam et al (1975) found elevated levels in patients presenting with subacute venous thrombosis. Stewart et al (1983) described significantly higher levels of platelet-specific proteins in patients with transient cerebral ischaemia, and

Handin et al (1978) found elevated levels in patients following myocardial infarction. Cella et al (1979) found elevated β-thromboglobulin levels in patients with peripheral vascular disease but not in patients with cerebro-vascular disease. Platelet-specific protein levels have been compared in diabetics with and without clinical evidence of vascular disease (Betteridge et al, 1981), and although there was a more pronounced increase in diabetics with retinopathy, those diabetics without clinical evidence of vascular disease still had higher levels of platelet-specific proteins than controls suggesting that the enhanced platelet activation may not just be a consequence of vascular damage but may precede its development.

So far elevated levels of platelet-specific proteins have been discussed purely as a likely measure of enhanced *in vivo* platelet-release reaction in diabetic subjects. However, do these platelet-specific proteins have a physiological role in their own right? The important platelet mitogen, platelet-derived growth factor which is an α-granule constituent along with β-thromboglobulin and platelet factor 4 has been discussed earlier in this chapter. Both β-thromboglobulin and platelet factor 4 have antiheparin activity. However, it is doubtful whether this property of the platelet-specific proteins has any physiological importance, since the concentration of heparin is probably insignificant (Niewiarowski & Paul, 1981). Nevertheless, these proteins also react with other glycosaminoglycans such as heparin sulphate (Barber et al, 1972; Niewiarowski et al, 1979). Heparin sulphate occurs on the surface of many cells including endothelial cells (Lindahl & Hook, 1978) and there is evidence that both platelet factor 4 (Busch et al, 1980) and β-thromboglobulin (Hope et al, 1979) bind to cultured endothelial cells. In addition, β-thromboglobulin appears to inhibit prostacyclin synthesis in bovine aortic endothelial cells (Hope et al, 1979). Platelet factor 4 appears to act as an inhibitor of collagenase which suggests a possible physiological role in connective tissue metabolism (Hiti-Harper et al, 1978). However, the possible physiological roles for β-thromboglobulin and platelet factor 4 remain to be determined.

Platelet prostaglandin and thromboxane production

As discussed previously, prostaglandins, thromboxanes and their precursor arachidonic acid are critical substances in platelet metabolism (Samuelsson, 1977), and there have been several studies of the activity of the prostaglandin pathway and thromboxane synthesis in platelets from diabetic subjects. Halushka et al (1977) demonstrated that diabetic platelets synthesised greater amounts of prostaglandin E_2 in response to various agonists compared to platelets from matched control subjects. Most of the patients studied were free of clinically detectable vascular disease. Subsequently, increased serum concentrations of the prostaglandins PGE_2 and $PGF_{1\alpha}$ were demonstrated in the serum of diabetic children (Chase et al, 1979). Although the findings indicated increased activity of the platelet prostaglandin pathway in diabetic subjects, they did not explain the increased platelet aggregation as these prostaglandins are not in themselves aggregatory.

The formation of the potent aggregating substance thromboxane A_2 in diabetic platelets has to be assessed indirectly because it is very labile with a half-life of approximately 30 seconds in aqueous solution (Hamberg et al, 1975). Malondialdehyde is a stable product of the conversion of endoperoxides to thromboxane A_2 by the microsomal enzyme thromboxane synthetase and is formed in equimolar amounts (Diczfalusy et al, 1977). Stuart et al (1979) showed that platelets obtained from pregnant diabetic women synthesised increased amounts of malondialdehyde. In addition, Betteridge et al (1981) found increased synthesis of malondialdehyde in washed platelets stimulated by arachidonic acid in 23 insulin-dependent and 25 non-insulin-dependent diabetics (20 males, 28 females) compared to 30 control subjects. Forty-one per cent of these diabetics had levels of malondialdehyde formation greater than the highest result seen in the control group, and this difference was highly significant (Betteridge et al, 1981).

Thromboxane A_2 formation has also been assessed by the measurement of thromboxane B_2 by radioimmunoassay. Thromboxane A_2 spontaneously rearranges to form thromboxane B_2 which is stable and considerably less potent (Friedman et al, 1979). Several studies have shown that diabetic platelets synthesise increased amounts of thromboxane A_2 as assessed by thromboxane B_2 levels (Ziboh et al, 1979; Butkus et al, 1980; Lagarde et al, 1980; Halushka et al, 1981b). Butkus et al (1980) measured thromboxane B_2 generation in response to exogenous arachidonic acid quantitated by electron-capture gas chromatography in a group of 180 insulin-dependent subjects. Although platelet thromboxane generation was elevated in diabetics without clinical evidence of vascular disease, the difference did not reach statistical significance. However, those diabetics with retinopathy, neuropathy, nephropathy, peripheral vascular disease or coronary vascular disease did show significantly enhanced platelet thromboxane generation compared to controls (Butkus et al, 1980). Ziboh et al (1979) also found that diabetics with complications had higher platelet thromboxane generation than diabetics without complications. However, in the study of Halushka et al (1981 b) thromboxane generation appeared to be increased in diabetics without complications, and evidence of increased thromboxane generation comes from studies using experimental animals, for instance the spontaneously diabetic BB–Wistar rat (Subbiah & Deitemeyer, 1980) and the streptozotocin diabetic rat (Johnson et al, 1980). In addition, a recent study has assessed platelet thromboxane production in insulin-dependent diabetics with and without coronary artery disease (Butkus et al, 1982). Platelets from diabetics with coronary artery disease had higher thromboxane production than those without coronary disease and platelets from diabetics in general produced more thromboxane than those from non-diabetics. However, those non-diabetics with

coronary disease showed high thromboxane production (Butkus et al, 1982).

Prostacyclin

The discovery of this highly important cyclo-oxygenation product of arachidonic acid, which is the most potent endogenous anti-platelet aggregatory agent known (Moncada et al, 1976 a), has stimulated interest in the possible effects of the diabetic state on its metabolism. Harrison et al (1978) found decreased prostacyclin production in aortic rings taken from severe streptozotocin diabetic rats. This original observation has been confirmed and extended by other workers. Silberbauer et al (1980) induced a mild form of diabetes in Göttingen miniature pigs by repeated administration of streptozotocin. The amount of prostacyclin generated (assayed by inhibition of ADP-induced aggregation) by vascular tissue was significantly reduced in these mildly diabetic animals (Silberbauer et al, 1980). The time-course of development of reduced vascular prostacyclin production was studied by El Tahir et al (1982). Although there was a slight reduction in aortic prostacyclin production in acutely diabetic rats (diabetic for up to 15 days), the differences were not statistically significant. However, in chronically diabetic rats (diabetic for eight weeks) vascular prostacyclin was markedly reduced (El Tahir et al, 1982).

The reduced production of vascular prostacyclin in chronically diabetic rats studied by Harrison et al (1980) was restored to normal by chronic (eight days) but not acute insulin treatment. This suggests that low prostacyclin production may be a consequence of arterial endothelial cell loss or damage and this requires restoration by normalisation of metabolism for some days before prostacyclin production returns to normal (Harrison et al, 1980).

It is obviously difficult to study arterial prostacyclin production in diabetic subjects. However, in a small study of vascular tissue removed at operation prostacyclin generation was found to be reduced in tissue from diabetics

(Johnson et al, 1979). Furthermore, Silberbauer et al (1979) showed that vein biopsies obtained from insulin-dependent diabetics generated significantly less prostacyclin compared to age- and sex-matched controls. On the other hand, Davis et al (1981) found that venous prostacyclin production was lower in a small group of diabetics with nil or minimal retinopathy compared to diabetics with proliferative retinopathy. This finding, albeit in very small numbers, would seem to suggest that reduced prostacyclin production may not have a role in the development of microvascular disease. However, it is likely that this finding may indicate increased prostacyclin production in response to vascular injury (Dollery et al, 1983).

Attempts have been made to measure plasma prostacyclin levels indirectly by radioimmunoassay measurement of 6-keto-PGF$_1\alpha$, a stable metabolite of prostacyclin. Using this method conflicting findings have been reported in studies of diabetic subjects (Dollery et al, 1979; Davis et al, 1981), and it is now generally accepted that there may be considerable non-specific interference in assaying this metabolite in plasma which might explain the different findings (Greaves & Preston, 1982; Dollery et al, 1983).

Two recent studies have examined the effect of the diabetic environment on prostacyclin production by cultured human endothelial cells (Paton et al, 1982 a; Patel et al, 1983). When these cells were incubated with serum from diabetic patients prostacyclin production was inhibited. The nature of the inhibitory factor or factors in the diabetic serum is not understood, but a likely contender would be lipid peroxides which are known to inhibit prostacyclin production and to be elevated in diabetic plasma.

In addition to the findings that vascular prostacyclin production may be decreased in diabetes, it has been shown that platelets obtained from diabetic subjects show diminished sensitivity to the antiaggregatory effects of prostacyclin *in vitro*. (Onodera et al, 1981; Betteridge et al, 1982; Jones et al, 1985). The pathogenesis of this finding is not known but it appears to be unrelated to any effect of the

diabetic state on platelet prostacyclin receptors as prostacyclin binding appears to be normal in diabetic platelets (Shepherd et al, 1983).

Platelet Function and Diabetic Control

The overall effect of diabetic control on platelet function remains to be clarified. Studies in this field are difficult to interpret due to the inherent variability of the measurements of platelet function. In addition, sample timing in relation to metabolic control in diabetic patients may be crucial. Hypoglycaemia, as might be expected, may affect platelet function substantially (Hutton et al, 1979; Hilsted et al, 1980), presumably by stimulating the release of counter-regulatory hormones, particularly adrenaline which is known to be a potent stimulus for platelet aggregation. Thus platelet aggregation induced by ADP *in vitro* was enhanced following hypoglycaemia and this was associated with a fall in platelet count (Hilsted et al, 1980). More recently, β-thromboglobulin has been shown to rise markedly during controlled hypoglycaemia in a group of insulin-dependent diabetics (Monnier et al, 1984). This latter finding provides further evidence of the *in vivo* platelet activation and release reaction. Therefore it is apparent that possible stimulation of platelet function by hypoglycaemia must be borne in mind when interpreting the results of longitudinal studies of 'tight' glycaemic control on platelet function. Hypoglycaemia may be asymptomatic (Calabrese et al, 1982) but still lead to secretion of adrenaline (Rizza et al, 1979) and hence activation of platelets. In addition, if samples for platelet function studies are taken from diabetic subjects during episodes of metabolic decompensation leading to diabetic ketoacidosis or the non-ketotic hyperosmolar syndrome, then platelet aggregation and consumption may be stimulated (Kwaan et al, 1972; Paton, 1981). As well as these acute metabolic derangements found in diabetes producing acute effects on platelet function, other factors known to influence platelet function in non-diabetics may be operative in the diabetic population under study, such as the presence of vascular disease, ingestion of aspirin-like substances, exercise, smoking, and the use of the contraceptive pill.

For these reasons studies detailing the effects of diabetic control on platelet function must be interpreted with caution. More work is needed in this area along with more reliable, reproducible and physiological assessments of platelet activity. In addition, it is important to know which of the altered plasma factors in the diabetic state are responsible for enhanced platelet function. If 'tight' diabetic control leads to restoration of platelet function to normal, is this a reflection of the fall in blood glucose, alteration in plasma lipids and fatty acids, restoration of normal endothelial cell integrity or other mechanisms? However, bearing in mind these constraints; what is the current evidence linking diabetic control and platelet function?

Associations between glycaemic control and parameters of platelet function have been sought both in cross-sectional studies and prospective studies and conflicting findings have been reported.

Platelet-specific proteins

In an early study of β-thromboglobulin in a mixed group of 72 diabetic subjects no correlation was found with simultaneous measurements of plasma glucose concentration (Burrows et al, 1978). Platelet factor 4 showed a significant positive correlation with plasma glucose concentration in a small group of insulin-dependent diabetics but no correlation was seen for β-thromboglobulin and no relationship was found for either of the platelet-specific proteins in a larger group of non-insulin-dependent diabetics (Davi et al, 1982). Several studies have sought relationships between glycosylated haemoglobin as a measure of overall glycaemic control and platelet-specific protein levels but no correlations were found (Mathews et al, 1979; Betteridge et al, 1981; Davi et al, 1982).

Equally conflicting results with regard to glycaemic control and platelet-specific protein levels have been reported in longitudinal studies. In nine newly diagnosed non-insulin-dependent diabetics mean β-thromboglobulin levels fell from 74 ng/ml (range 24–177 ng/ml) to 39 ng/ml as treatment with diet and hypoglycaemic agents reduced mean blood glucose concentrations from 14.3 to 8.5 mmol/l. (Preston et al, 1978). However, in longitudinal studies of moderately well controlled insulin-dependent diabetics treated with CS11 for two weeks (Delamothe & Betteridge, 1985) or four to eight weeks (Rosove et al, 1984) which led to significant lowering of mean plasma glucose and glycosylated haemoglobin levels, no changes were observed in platelet factor 4 or β-thromboglobulin levels. On the other hand, in a short-term study using the artificial pancreas, normalisation of blood glucose for 48 hours led to a significant fall in β-thromboglobulin levels (Voisin et al, 1983).

As has been discussed elsewhere in this book, hyperlipoproteinaemia is common in diabetes mellitus and in some studies correlations have been sought between platelet-specific protein levels and fasting total serum cholesterol, triglycerides and the individual lipoproteins. These measurements were available in 49 of the diabetic subjects studied by Betteridge et al (1981). Small but statistically significant correlations were found between β-thromboglobulin levels and total triglyceride, VLDL-triglyceride, LDL-cholesterol and HDL/total cholesterol ratio. The correlations were positive apart from the correlation with HDL/total cholesterol which was negative. These findings suggest that changes seen in platelet-specific proteins in diabetes might be secondary to associated hyperlipoproteinaemia. In addition, these correlations between individual lipid and lipoprotein concentrations and platelet-specific proteins may explain the changes of platelet-specific proteins with instigation of diabetic therapy (Preston et al, 1978), as lipid levels would be expected to be elevated in uncontrolled diabetes and to fall with improved control (Paisey et al,

1978; Simpson et al, 1979). This suggested association between lipid and lipoprotein levels and enhanced platelet function in diabetes is supported by many studies which have described abnormal platelet function in hyperlipidaemic non-diabetic subjects (Nordoy & Rodset, 1971; Carvalho et al, 1974; Shattil et al, 1977; Colman, 1978; Joist et al, 1979; Tremoli et al, 1979) which have measured *in vitro* platelet aggregation, platelet factor 4, plasma antiheparin activity and a bleeding-time test. In addition, the platelet-specific proteins β-thromboglobulin and platelet factor 4 were highly significantly elevated in a large group of hyperlipaemic subjects compared to normolipaemic controls (Zahavi et al, 1981).

The mechanism of lipid-induced effects of platelet function has received considerable attention. Shattil et al (1975) studied the effect of incubating normal platelets with cholesterol-rich liposomes. This led to a substantial increase in platelet cholesterol concentration, the bulk of this increase being associated with the platelet membrane. Along with these changes in cholesterol concentration the cholesterol-rich platelets showed enhanced sensitivity to adrenaline and ADP measured by aggregometry and ^{14}C-serotonin release. Conversely, platelets incubated with 'cholesterol-poor' liposomes showed a reduced cholesterol content and significantly reduced sensitivity to ADP. On the basis of these findings, Shattil et al (1975) postulated that cholesterol enrichment of the platelet membrane might affect the membrane fluidity and consequently the sensitivity to aggregating agonists. In support of this suggestion the same workers (Shattil et al, 1977) found that platelets from patients with Type 2 hyperlipoproteinaemia had a higher cholesterol/phospholipid ratio and other workers have found an elevated platelet-free cholesterol in patients with the same condition (Miettinen, 1974). In addition, Shattil and Cooper (1976) described increased platelet membrane microviscosity following incubation of platelets with 'cholesterol-rich' liposomes and Sinha et al (1977) found an impaired response of the membrane-associated enzyme adenylate cyclase to the stimulating effect of various agents including prostaglandin E_1 as shown by a decrease in production of cyclic AMP. More recent studies have demonstrated that increases in the cholesterol/phospholipid ratio of platelets resulted in increased liberation of arachidonate (Wörner & Patscheke, 1980). In addition, Aviram and Brook (1983) have provided evidence for a direct effect on *in vitro* platelet function for the cholesterol-rich lipoprotein, LDL and the triglyceride-rich lipoprotein, VLDL. These workers incubated the purified lipoprotein for 30 minutes with gel-filtered platelets and demonstrated that VLDL and LDL increased thrombin-induced platelet aggregation and ^{14}C-serotonin release induced by adrenaline ADP and thrombin. However, Hassall et al (1983), who examined the relationship of *in vitro* aggregation to adrenaline, ADP, collagen and thrombin to prevailing .lipid and lipoprotein concentrations in a normal male population, found little relationship between VLDL and platelet sensitivity except for a reduced adrenaline response in subjects in the lowest quintile for VLDL concentrations. In contrast, total and LDL cholesterol concentrations did appear to influence platelet sensitivity to adrenaline and to a lesser extent ADP (Hassall et al, 1983).

Lipoproteins may indirectly affect platelet function by altering vascular endothelial cell function. Recent experimental work has suggested that lipoproteins (VLDL) obtained from diabetic animals (streptozotocin diabetic rats) may be more toxic to cultured porcine endothelial cells than lipoproteins obtained from control animals. This effect which may be due to increased lipid peroxide levels in diabetes was reversed by insulin treatment (Arbogast et al, 1982). Other studies have shown increased lipid peroxide levels in lipoproteins isolated from diabetic patients (Nishigaki et al, 1981) and animals (Higuchi, 1982). These findings suggest that lipoprotein abnormalities in the diabetic state may also indirectly affect platelet function by damaging vascular endothelium. There is as yet no direct measure of endothelial damage in the intact animal. However, some recent studies have measure plasma levels of Factor VIII-related antigen as an indirect measure of endothelial cell damage together with β-thromboglobulin levels. Rak et al (1983) found that plasma levels of both proteins were elevated in diabetics including children. It is difficult to determine therefore whether endothelial damage preceded the evidence of enhanced platelet-release reaction or not. Janka et al (1983) studied Factor VIII-related antigen and β-thromboglobulin levels in groups of diabetics with and without vascular disease. These authors found an increase in Factor VIII-related antigen in all groups of diabetics whereas β-thromboglobulin was only elevated in diabetics with retinopathy. This study suggests that endothelial damage (as assessed by Factor VIII-related antigen levels) may precede evidence of *in vivo* platelet aggregation. Recently, Winocour et al (1983) have been able to examine the time-course of alterations in platelet function and vascular endothelial cell damage as assessed by measurement of plasma levels of von Willebrand Factor and Factor VIII-related antigen in rats made diabetic with streptozotocin. These authors found that whereas enhanced platelet function (increased aggregation to ADP) was detectable as early as three days following induction of diabetes, elevated levels of the Factor VIII components were not seen for 14–28 days. Therefore, these findings suggest that in this experimental model evidence of enhanced platelet function occurs before evidence of endothelial damage, suggesting that the enhanced platelet aggregation is not merely secondary to endothelial cell damage. In this study no difference was observed in the plasma cholesterol concentration between control and diabetic rats. However, plasma triglycerides were elevated in the diabetic animals soon after the induction of the disease and the authors speculated that this may have contributed to the development of the platelet and vessel-wall changes.

Platelet aggregation

The relationship between platelet aggregation and diabetic control is even more confounding than that for the platelet-specific proteins, various studies either showing no change, increased or decreased platelet aggregation in response to improved glycaemic control. Platelet aggregation in response to adrenaline showed striking changes when studied before and after stabilisation of poorly controlled diabetics (Peterson et al, 1977) in that the lag phase following the addition of adrenaline was prolonged from a mean of 19 to 65 seconds following stabilisation. In addition, there was a significant inverse correlation between glycosylated haemoglobin levels and the lag phase, suggesting that the platelets were less sensitive to adrenaline when better glycaemic control had been achieved (Peterson et al, 1977). More recently, platelet-aggregation responses have been studied in diabetics treated with CS11 or the artificial pancreas. After strict metabolic control was achieved in 10 insulin-dependent diabetics for 24 hours with the aid of the artificial pancreas, mean blood glucose levels falling from 13.3 mmol/l to 5.1 mmol/l, a significant decrease in the aggregation response to ADP, was observed (Giugliano et al, 1982). Along with this there was a significant reduction in circulating platelet aggregates. No such changes were observed in a group of eight insulin-dependent diabetics whose glycaemic control was only monitored during the study period (Giugliano et al, 1982). Other authors found similar findings with regard to circulating platelet aggregates. A group of 92 diabetics were divided into 39 with poor control (glycosylated haemoglobin >9 per cent) and 53 with good control (glycosylated haemoglobin <9 per cent) and the results of the platelet-aggregate ratio analysed. Diabetics with poor control had platelet-aggregate ratios significantly lower than those with good control, indicating the presence of more circulating aggregates in the poorly controlled group. In addition, a significant inverse correlation between the platelet-aggregate ratio and glycosylated haemoglobin was found for the whole group (Dettori et al, 1983).

Juhan et al (1982) also studied the effect of glycaemic normalisation by the artificial pancreas on platelet function but employed other techniques. These authors attempted to assess platelet function in citrated whole blood by determining the platelet aggregates formed following electromagnetic agitation for 15 minutes. The aggregates formed were fixed with formol and the results expressed as the percentage of platelets aggregated compared to a reference platelet count performed before the agitation. After 24 hours of normoglycaemia platelet aggregation returned to levels seen in non-diabetic controls (Juhan et al, 1982). Using CS11 to obtain improved glycaemic control for longer periods other workers have failed to demonstrate changes in platelet aggregation *in vitro* (Rosove et al, 1984; Delamothe & Betteridge, 1985). However, one study has not only shown persistence of enhanced platelet reactivity in response to collagen and sodium arachidonate despite a 16-week period of near normal glycaemic control but also an increase in platelet reactivity to ADP (Jackson et al, 1984).

Thromboxane

Thromboxane production by platelets stimulated with arachidonic acid showed a significant positive correlation with the fasting plasma glucose concentration obtained at the same time in a group of 15 diabetics studied by Halushka et al (1981 b). In addition, platelet thromboxane synthesis was lower in a group of diabetics treated with CS11 for six months compared to a control group on conventional therapy (McDonald et al, 1982). However, when normal platelets were incubated with increasing glucose concentrations *in vitro* thromboxane production was unaffected (Best et al, 1979), and the findings of Halushka et al (1981 b) and McDonald et al (1982) have not been supported by a recent study of platelet thromboxane generation before and after CS11 (Jackson et al, 1984). These authors measured thromboxane generation in response to arachidonic acid and collagen in a group of 11 diabetic patients with neuropathy. Before CS11, arachidonic acid-stimulated thromboxane production was enhanced in the diabetics compared

to controls and this enhanced production persisted after CS11 for 16 weeks. On the other hand, collagen-stimulated thromboxane production was similar to controls before CS11 apart from at the lowest collagen concentration (0.5 μg/ml) when thromboxane production was in fact lower than that seen in control subjects. After CS11 this apparent subnormal thromboxane production returned to normal (Jackson et al, 1984). This finding may be due to a reduced level of arachidonic acid in platelet membrane phospholipids of diabetic subjects as described by Jones et al (1983). This reduced level of arachidonic acid showed a negative correlation with glycosylated haemoglobin (Jones et al, 1983). The finding therefore of an increase in collagen-stimulated thromboxane production by CS11 could be explained by an increased availability of arachidonic acid from membrane phospholipids (Jackson et al, 1984).

Prostacyclin

Information about the effect of diabetic control on prostacyclin production comes from animal studies. Harrison et al (1980) demonstrated that the reduced prostacyclin release (measured by bioassay) from aorta and renal cortex of streptozotocin-induced diabetic rats was restored to that seen in control non-diabetic rats by chronic (eight days) treatment with insulin. However, no effects were seen on prostacyclin production acutely after the start of insulin treatment. It is likely that chronic insulin treatment is necessary to allow endothelial cell loss or damage to be repaired (Harrison et al, 1980). These findings have been extended in the streptozotocin diabetic rat by Rogers and Larkins (1981). These authors measured the production of 6-oxo-prostaglandin $F_1\alpha$, the stable metabolite of prostacyclin by rat aorta. They demonstrated that the reduced production of 6-oxo-prostaglandin $F_1\alpha$ seen in chronically diabetic rats (four-six weeks) could be restored by a dose of insulin (8 U/kg/day) that only partially corrected their plasma glucose and body weight (Rogers & Larkins, 1981).

The studies discussed so far have dealt with the effects of insulin deficiency in the experimental diabetic rat on prostacyclin production and the effects of insulin treatment. However, the possible role of peripheral hyperinsulinaemia as a risk factor for vascular disease has been emphasised (Stout, 1981), and pertinent to this hypothesis are the findings of Lasche and Larson (1982). These authors studied the effects of high insulin concentrations on prostacyclin production by rat aortic rings *in vitro* and demonstrated that prostacyclin production was significantly reduced in the presence of insulin at concentrations of 2500, 500 and 250 μU/ml (Lasche & Larson, 1982). Thus a possible deleterious effect of hyperinsulinaemia may be the inhibition of prostacyclin production by arterial wall.

The sensitivity of platelets from diabetic subjects to the antiaggregatory effects of prostacyclin has been examined in a cross-sectional study using the electronic whole blood platelet aggregometer (Jones et al, 1985). A positive correlation was found between glycosylated haemoglobin concentration and the prostacyclin concentration necessary to inhibit ADP-induced platelet aggregation by 50 per cent. This finding suggests that under situations of poor glycaemic control platelets from diabetic subjects are less sensitive to the antiaggregatory effects of prostacyclin (Jones et al, 1985).

Sulphonylureas and Other Agents

There are a variety of sulphonylurea agents available for the therapy of diet-failed non-insulin-dependent diabetic subjects, varying mainly in their half-life and mode of excretion. In addition to their hypoglycaemic action it is probable that some or all of these compounds may have antiplatelet effects. Thus gliclazide depresses various parameters of platelet function *in vitro* and appears to inhibit arachidonate release from platelet phospholipids (Tsuboi et al, 1981) and to activate platelet adenylate cyclase leading to increased levels of cyclic AMP (Lagarde et al, 1975). In addition, *ex vivo* platelet

aggregation to ADP and adrenaline was significantly reduced in diabetic subjects treated for up to a year with therapeutic doses of gliclazide (Poari et al, 1979). These authors considered that the antiplatelet action observed was unrelated to effects on glycaemic control as the two effects were dissociated in time (Poari et al, 1979). However, other workers who studied the effect of gliclazide in diabetic subjects have felt that the beneficial effects of gliclazide on platelet function were likely to be due to its hypoglycaemic action rather than to any direct effect on haemostatic function (Paton et al, 1982 b).

Gliclazide is the sulphonylurea that has received most study in terms of possible effects on platelet function. However, other sulphonylurea preparations may also have antiplatelet effects. Thus tolbutamide in high concentrations has been shown to inhibit platelet aggregation and interfere with the platelet-release reaction (Roth et al, 1971). In addition, in a study of diet, diet plus glibenclamide and diet plus gliclazide on plasma glucose and platelet function in a group of newly diagnosed non-insulin-dependent diabetics, both glibenclamide and gliclazide reduced the increased platelet sensitivity to ADP seen in the diet period (Klaff et al, 1979). Furthermore, glibenclamide therapy was associated with a significant reduction in the platelet-aggregation response to adrenaline (10 μmol) and collagen (750 μg/ml). Obviously further work needs to be done in this area, and long-term studies now in progress using antiplatelet agents such as aspirin and dipyridamole need to be evaluated for possible protective effects on the development of microvascular and macrovascular disease in diabetic subjects. In addition, the newer agents such as prostacyclin and its stable analogues and thromboxane synthetase inhibitors need to be similarly evaluated. Certainly a thromboxane synthetase inhibitor has been shown to reduce urinary albumin excretion in insulin-dependent diabetics (Barnett et al, 1984). A further potentially exciting area yet to be explored in the diabetic population is the dietary substitution of the ω-3 series of fatty acids such as eicosapentaenoic and decosahexaenoic acids which has been shown to favourably affect platelet function in non-diabetic subjects (Siess et al, 1980; Thorngren & Gustafson, 1981; Lorenz et al, 1983).

Conclusions

In this chapter I have described some aspects of platelet physiology and biochemistry and the possible role of this interesting cell in the pathogenesis of atherosclerosis and thrombosis. A tentative conclusion that could be drawn from the discussion of platelet-function abnormalities in diabetics would be that the increased platelet reactivity may represent a prethrombotic state and contribute to the as-yet-unexplained increased vascular risk in these patients.

However, although there have been tremendous developments in this field there remain many unanswered questions. As knowledge of basic platelet metabolism increases it will be more easy to identify platelet abnormalities and their pathogenesis in diabetes mellitus. Future developments hopefully will lead to better and more reliable tests of platelet function able to establish the prethrombotic state with more certainty. This would enable prospective studies to be performed to determine the importance of platelet function in the development of vascular disease. In addition, improved therapeutic agents with more specific and controlled effects on platelet metabolism may be developed allowing more effective intervention. Certainly two recent preliminary reports of prospective studies of currently available antiplatelet agents and the progression of vascular disease in diabetics have been disappointing (Abraira et al, 1985; Kohner & Baudoin, 1985).

The effects of the diabetic state on the vascular endothelium and its interaction with platelets and other formed elements of blood need to be explored, which will require specific measurements of *in vivo* endothelial cell metabolism. In addition, the role of the numerous growth factors and their control in platelets, macrophages and endothelium needs to be explored in diabetes and should lead to new insights in the development of diabetic vascular complications.

References

Abraira, C., Colwell, J.A., Bingham, S.F. et al (1985). The VA Cooperative Society Group. *Diabet. Res. Clin. Pract.* Suppl. 1, S3.

Adelstein, R.S. and Pollard, R.D. (1978). Platelet contractile proteins. *Prog. Hemost. Thromb.* **4**, 37–58.

Aiken, J.W., Gormon, R.R. and Shebuski, R.J. (1979). Prevention of blockage of partially obstructed coronary arteries with prostacyclin correlates with inhibition of platelet aggregation. *Prostaglandins* **17**, 483–494.

Allan, D. and Mitchell, R.H. (1979). In Hopkins, C.R. and Duncan, C.J. (eds), *Secretory Mechanisms. S.E.B. Symposium 33*, Cambridge, Cambridge University Press, pp. 323–336.

Arbogast, B.W., Lee G.M. and Raymond, T.L. (1982). *In vitro* injury of porcine aortic endothelial cells by very-low-density lipoproteins from diabetic rat serum. *Diabetes* **31**, 593–599.

Armstrong, J.M., Lattimer, N., Moncada, S. et al (1978). Comparison of the vasodepressor effects of prostacyclin and 6-oxo-prostaglandin $F_{1\alpha}$ with those of prostaglandin E_2 in rats and rabbits. *Br. J. Pharmacol.* **62**, 125–130.

Aviram, M. and Brook, J.G. (1983). The effect of blood constituents on platelet function: role of blood cells and plasma lipoproteins. *Artery* **11**, 297–305.

Badawi, H., El-Sawy, M. and Mikhail, M. (1970). Platelets, coagulation and fibrinolysis in diabetic and non-diabetic patients with quiescent coronary heart disease. *Angiology* **21**, 511–519.

Barber, A.G., Kaser-Glanzmann, R., Jakabova, M. et al (1972). Characterization of chondroitin sulphate proteoglycan carrier for heparin neutrilizing activity (PF_4) released from human blood platelets. *Biochim. Biophys. Acta* **286**, 312–329.

Barnett, A.H., Wakelin, K., Leatherdale, B.A. et al (1984). Specific thromboxane synthetase inhibition and albumin excretion rate in insulin-dependent diabetes. *Lancet* **i**, 1322–1325.

Bayer, B-L., Blass, K-E. and Forster, W. (1979). Anti-aggregatory effect of prostacyclin (PGI_2) *in vivo. Br. J. Pharmacol.* **66**, 10–12.

Behnke, O. (1970). The morphology of blood platelet membrane systems. *Ser. Haematol.* **3**, 3–16.

Bell, R.L., Kennerly, D.N., Stanford, N. et al (1979). Diglyceride lipase: a pathway for arachidonate release from human platelets. *Proc. Natl. Acad. Sci. USA* **76**, 3238–3241.

Benevist, J., Henson, P.M. and Cochrane, C.G. (1972). Leucocyte dependent histamine release from rabbit platelets: the role of IgE, basophils and a platelet activating factor. *J. Exp. Med.* **136**, 1356–1377.

Bennett, J.S. and Vilaire, G. (1979). Exposure of platelet fibrinogen receptors by ADP and epinephrine. *J. Clin. Invest.* **64**, 1393–1401.

Bensoussan, D., Levy-Toledano, S., Passa, P. et al (1975). Platelet hyperaggregation and increased plasma level of von Willebrand factor in diabetics with retinopathy. *Diabetologia* **11**, 307–312.

Berndt, M.C. and Phillips, D.R. (1981). Platelet membrane proteins: composition and receptor function. In Gordon, J.L. (ed.), *Platelets in Biology and Pathology 2* Oxford, Elsevier/North Holland, pp. 43–75.

Bergvist, D. and Arfos, K.E. (1976). Microvascular haemostasis and the effect of local stimulation and inhibition of platelet function. An experimental study in rabbits. *Thromb. Haemost.* **45**, 150–153.

Best, L.C., Jones, P.B. and Preston, N.E. (1979). Effect of glucose on platelet thromboxane biosynthesis. *Lancet* **ii**, 790.

Betteridge, D.J., El Tahir, K.E.H., Reckless, J.P.D. et al (1982). Platelets from diabetic subjects show diminished sensitivity to prostacyclin. *Eur. J. Clin. Invest.* **12**, 395–398.

Betteridge, D.J., Zahavi, J., Jones, N.A.G. et al (1981). Platelet function in diabetes mellitus in relationship to complications, glycosylated haemoglobin and serum lipoproteins. *Eur. J. Clin. Invest.* **11**, 273–277.

Blackwell, G.J., Flower, R.J., Russell-Smith, N. et al (1978). Prostacyclin is produced in whole blood. *Br. J. Pharmacol.* **64**, p. 436.

Born, G.V.R. (1962). Aggregation of blood platelets by adenosine diphosphate and its reversal. *Nature* **194**, 927–929.

Born, G.V.R. (1983). Platelets in atherogenesis and thrombogenesis. In Miller, N.E. (ed.), *Atherosclerosis: Mechanisms and Approaches to Therapy*, New York, Raven Press, pp. 45–53.

Born, G.V.R. and Cross, M.J. (1964). Effects of inorganic ions and of plasma proteins on the aggregation of blood platelets by adenosine diphosphate. *J. Physiol.* (London), **170**, 397–414.

Bornstein, P. and Sage, H. (1980). Structurally distinct collagen types. *Am. Rev. Biochem.* **49**, 957–1003.

Bouch, D.C. and Montgomery, D.L. (1970). Cardiac lesions in fatal cases of recent myocardial ischaemia from a coronary care unit. *Br. Heart. J.* **32**, 795–803.

Boullin, D.J., Bunting, S., Blaso, W.P. et al (1979). Responses of human and baboon arteries to prostaglandin endoperoxides and biologically generated and synthetic prostacyclin: their relevance to cerebral arterial spasm in man. *Br. J. Clin. Pharmacol.* **7**, 129–147.

Bowen-Pope, D.F. and Ross, R. (1984). Platelet-derived growth factor. *Clin. Endocrinol. Metab.* **13**, 191–205.

Brinkhaus, K.M., Read, M.S. and Mason, R.G. (1965). Plasma thrombocyte-agglutinating activity and fibrinogen. Synergism with adenosine diphosphate. *Lab. Invest.* **14**, 335–342.

Brooks, C.J.W., Steel, G., Gilbert, J.D. et al (1971). Lipids of human atheroma. 4. Characterisations of a new group of polar sterol esters from human atherosclerotic plaques. *Atherosclerosis* **13**, 223–237.

Bunting, S., Moncada, S. and Vane, J.R. (1983). The prostacyclin–thromboxane balance: pathophysiological and therapeutic implications. *Br. Med. Bull.* **39**, 271–276.

Buonassisi, V. (1973). Sulphated mucopolysaccharide synthesis and secretion in endothelial cell cultures. *Exp. Cell Res.* **76**, 363–368.

Burrows, A.W., Chavin, S. and Hockaday,T.D.R. (1978). Plasma β-thromboglobulin concentration in diabetes mellitus. *Lancet* **i**, 235–237.

Busch, C., Dawes, J., Pepper, D.S. et al (1980). Binding of platelet factor 4 to cultured human umbilical vein endothelial cells. *Thromb. Res.* **19**, 129–238.

Butkus, A., Shirey, E.K. and Schumaker, O.P. (1982). Thromboxane biosynthesis in platelets of diabetic and coronary artery disease patients. *Artery* **11**, 238–251.

Butkus, A., Srinska, V.A. and Schumaker, O.P. (1980). Thromboxane production and platelet aggregation in diabetic subjects with clinical complications. *Thromb. Res.* **19**, 211–223.

Calabrese, G., Bueti, A., Santeusanio, F. et al (1982). Continuous subcutaneous insulin infusion treatment in insulin-dependent diabetic patients: a comparison with conventional optimized treatment in a long term study. *Diabet. Care* **5**, 457–465.

Campbell, I.W., Dawes, J., Fraser, D.M. et al (1977). Plasma β-thromboglobulin in diabetes mellitus. *Diabetes* **26**, 1175–1177.

Cardinal, D.C. and Flower, R.J. (1980). The electronic aggregometer: a novel device for assessing platelet behaviour in blood. *J. Pharmacol. Methods.* **3**, 135–158.

Carey, F., Menashi, S. and Crawford, N. (1982). Localization of cyclo-oxygenase and thromboxane synthetase in human platelet intracellular membranes. *Biochem. J.* **204**, 847–851.

Carvalho, A.C.A., Colman, R.W. and Lees, R.S. (1974). Platelet function in hyperbetalipoproteinaemia. *New Engl. J. Med* **290**, 434–438.

Cella, G., Zahavi, J., De Haas, H.A. et al (1979). β-Thromboglobulin, platelet production time and platelet function in vascular disease. *Br. J. Haematol.* **43**, 127–136.

Chait, A., Ross, R., Albers, J.J. et al (1980). Platelet-derived growth factor stimulates activity of low density lipoprotein receptors. *Proc. Natl. Acad. Sci. USA* **77**, 4084–4088.

Chandler, A.B. and Hand, R.A. (1961). Phagocytized platelets: a source of lipids in human thrombi and atherosclerotic plaques. *Science* **134**, 946–947.

Chapman, I. (1965). Morphogenesis of occluding coronary thrombosis. *Arch. Pathol.* **80**, 256–261.

Chase, H.P., Williams, R.L. and Dupont, J. (1979). Increased prostaglandin synthesis in childhood diabetes mellitus. *J. Pediatr.* **94**, 185–189.

Chien, S. (1978). Transport across arterial endothelium. *Prog. Haemost. Thromb.* **4**, 1–36.

Chignard, M., Couedic, J.P., Tence, M. et al (1979). The role of platelet-activating factor in platelet aggregation. *Nature* **279**, 799–800.

Clemmons, M., van Wyk, J.J. and Pledger, W.J. (1980). Sequential addition of platelet factor and plasma to BALB/c3T3 fibroblast cultures stimulates somatomedin-C binding early in cell cycle. *Proc. Natl. Acad. Sci. USA* **77**, 6644–6648.

Cohen, I., Gerrard, J.M. and White, J.G. (1980). The role of contractile filaments in platelet activation. In Peeters, H. (ed.), *Proteins of the Biological Fluids*, New York, Pergamon Press, pp. 555–566.

Coker, S.J., Parratt, J.R., Ledingham, I.McA. and Zeitlin, I.J. (1981). Thromboxane and prostacyclin release from ischaemic myocardium in relation to arrhythmias. *Nature* **291**, 323–324.

Colman, R.W. (1978). Platelet function in hyperbetalipoproteinaemia. *Thromb. Haemost.* **39**, 284–293.

Colwell, J.A., Halushka, P.V., Sarki, K.E. et al (1978). Platelet function and diabetes mellitus. *Med. Clin. North Am.* **62**, 753–766.

Colwell, J.A., Winocour, P.D. and Halushka, P.V. (1983). Do platelets have anything to do with diabetic microvascular disease? *Diabetes* **32**, Suppl. 2, 14–19.

Constantinides, P. (1966). Plaque fissures in human coronary thrombosis. *J. Atheroscl. Res.* **6**, 1–17.

Corbella, E., Miragliotta, G., Masper, R. et al (1979). Platelet aggregation and antithrombin III levels in diabetic children. *Haemostasis* **8**, 30–37.

Crawford, M.A. (1983). Back to essential fatty acids and their prostanoid derivatives. *Br. Med. Bull.* **39**, 210–213.

Creter, D., Pavlotzky, F. and Savir, H. (1978). Platelet aggregation in diabetic retinopathy. *Acta Haematol. (Basel)* **60**, 53–55.

Cutler, L., Rodan, G. and Feinstein, M.G. (1978). Cytochemical localization of adenylate cyclase and of calcium ion, magnesium ion-activated ATP-ases in the dense tubular system of human blood platelets. *Biochim. Biophys. Acta* **542**, 357–371.

D'Angelo, V., Villa, S., Mysliwiec, M. et al (1978). Defective fibrinolytic and prostacyclin-like activity in human atheromatous plaques. *Thromb. Diath. Haemorrh.* **39**, 535–536.

Davi, G., Rini, G.B., Averna, M. et al (1982). Enhanced platelet release reaction in insulin-dependent and insulin-independent diabetic patients. *Haemostasis* **12**, 275–281.

Davies, M.J. and Thomas, T. (1981). The pathological basis and microanatomy of occlusive thrombus formation in human arteries. *Philos. Trans. R. Soc. Lond. [Biol] Sci.* **294**, 225–229.

Davies, P.F. and Ross, R. (1978). Mediation of pinocytosis in cultured arterial smooth muscle and endothelial cells by platelet-derived growth factor. *J. Cell Bio.* **79**, 663–671.

Davis, J.W., Hartman, C.R., Davies, R.F. et al (1982). Platelet aggregate ratio in diabetes mellitus. *Acta Haematol.* **67**, 222–224.

Davis, T.M.E., Brown, E., Finch, D.R. et al (1981). *In vitro* venous prostacyclin production, plasma 6-keto-prostaglandin $F_{1\alpha}$ concentrations and diabetic retinopathy. *Br. Med. J.* **282**, 1259–1262.

Davis, T.M.E., Mitchell, M.D. and Turner, R.C. (1979). Prostacyclin and thromboxane metabolites in diabetes. *Lancet* **ii**, 789–790.

Dawes, J., Smith, R.C. and Pepper, D.S. (1978). The release distribution and clearance of human β-thromboglobulin and platelet factor 4. *Thromb. Res.* **12**, 851–881.

Dawson, W., Boot, J.R., Cockerill, A.F. et al (1976). Release of novel prostaglandins and thromboxanes after immunological challenge. *Nature* **262**, 699–702.

Defreyn, G., Machin, S.J., Carreras, L.O. et al (1981). Familial bleeding tendency with partial platelet thromboxane synthetase deficiency: reorientation of cyclic endoperoxide metabolism. *Br. J. Haematol.* **49**, 29–41.

Dejana, E., Cazenave, J.P., Groves, H.M. et al (1980). The effect of aspirin inhibition of prostacyclin production on platelet adherence to normal and damaged rabbit aortae. *Thromb. Res.* **17**, 456–464.

Delamothe, A.P. and Betteridge, D.J. (1985). Continuous subcutaneous insulin infusion and risk factors for vascular disease. *Diabet. Med.* **2**, 219A.

Dembinska-Kiec, A., Gryglewski, T., Zmuda, A. et al (1977). The generation of prostacyclin by arteries and by coronary vascular bed is reduced in experimental atherosclerosis in rabbits. *Prostaglandins* **14**, 1025–1034.

Dettori, A.G., Quaintavalla, R. and Poli, T. (1983). Circulating platelet aggregates in diabetes mellitus. *Acta Haematol.* **96**, 65–66.

Deuel, T.F., Senior, R.M., Huang, J.S. et al (1982). Chemotaxis of monocytes and neutrophils to platelet derived growth factor. *J. Clin. Invest.* **69**, 1046–1049.

Diczfalusy, U., Falardeau, P. and Hammarstrom, S. (1977). Conversion of prostaglandin endoperoxides to C_{17}-hydroxyacids catalyzed by human platelet thromboxane synthase. *FEBS Lett.* **84**, 271–274.

Diczfalusy, U. and Hammarström, S. (1977). Inhibitors of thromboxane synthase in human platelets. *FEBS Lett.* **82**, 107–110.

Dollery, C.T., Barrow, S.E., Blair, I.A. et al (1983). Role of prostacyclin. In Miller, N.E. (ed.), *Atherosclerosis: Mechanisms and Approaches to Therapy*, New York, Raven Press, pp. 105–123.

Dollery, C.T., Friedman, L.A., Hensby, C.N. et al (1979). Circulating prostacyclin may be reduced in diabetes. *Lancet* **ii**, 1365.

Duguid, J.B. (1946). Thrombosis as a factor in the pathogenesis of coronary atherosclerosis. *J. Pathol.* **58**, 207–212.

Dusting, G.J., Chapple, D.J., Hughes, R. et al (1978). Prostacyclin (PGI_2) induces coronary vasodilatation in anaesthetised dogs. *Cardiovasc. Res.* **12**, 720–730.

Dusting, G.J., Moncada S. and Vane, J.R. (1979). Prostaglandins, their intermediates and precursors: cardiovascular actions and regulatory roles in normal and abnormal circulatory systems. *Prog. Cardiovasc. Dis.* **21**, 405–430.

Eldor, A., Falcone, D.J., Hajjar, D.P. et al (1981). Recovery of prostacyclin production by de-endothelialized rabbit aorta. Critical role of smooth muscle cells. *J. Clin. Invest.* **67**, 735–741.

Ellis, E.F., Wei, E.P. and Kontos, H.A. (1979). Vasodilation of cat cerebral arterioles by prostaglandins D_2, E_2, G_2 & I_2. *Am. J. Physiol.* **237**, H381–H385.

El-Maraghi, A. and Genton, E. (1980). The relevance of platelet and fibrin thromboembolism of the coronary microcirculation with special reference to sudden cardiac death. *Circulation* **62**, 936–944.

El Tahir, K.E.H., Williams, K.L. and Betteridge, D.J. (1982). The effect of experimental diabetes on prostaglandin production by tissues from pregnant rats. *Prostagland. Leukotr. Med.* **8**, 429–435.

Faggiotto, A. and Ross, R. (1984). Studies of hypercholesterolaemia in the non-human primate. *Arteriosclerosis* **4**, 341–356.

Faggiotto, A., Ross, R. and Harker, L. (1984). Studies of hypercholesterolaemia in the non-human primate. a. Changes that lead to fatty streak formation. *Arteriosclerosis* **4**, 323–338.

Feinstein, M.B. (1980). Release of intracellular membrane bound calcium precedes the onset of stimulus induced exocytosis in platelets. *Biochim. Biophys. Res. Commun.* **93**, 593–600.

Fitzgerald, G.A., Brash, A.R., Falardeau, P. et al (1981). Estimated rate of prostacyclin secretion into the circulation of normal man. *J. Clin. Invest.* **68**, 1272–1276.

Florentin, R.A., Nam, S.C., Lee, K.T. et al (1969). Increased ^{3}H-thymidine incorporation into endothelial cells of swine fed cholesterol for 3 days. *Exp. Mol. Pathol.* **1**, 250–255.

French, J.E. (1966). Atherosclerosis in relation to the structure and function of the arterial intima with special reference to the endothelium. *Int. Rev. Exp. Pathol.* **5**, 253–352.

Friedman, H. (1970). Pathogenesis of coronary thrombosis, intramural and intraluminal haemorrhage. In Halonen, L.A. (ed.), *Thrombosis and Coronary Heart Disease, Vol. 4*, Basel, Karger.

Friedman, L.S., Fitzpatrick, T.M., Bloom, M.D. et al (1979). Cardiovascular and pulmonary effects of thromboxane B_2 in the dog. *Circ. Res.* **44**, 748–751.

Gaarder, A., Jonsen, J., Laland, S. et al (1961). Adenosine diphosphate in red cells as a factor in the adhesiveness of human blood platelets. *Nature* **192**, 531–532.

Garcia, M.J., McNamara, P.M., Gordon, T. et al (1974). Morbidity and mortality in diabetics in the Framingham Population, Sixteen-year follow up study. *Diabetes* **23**, 105–111.

Gartner, T.K., Phillips, D.R. and Williams, D.C. (1980). Expression of thrombin-enhanced platelet lectin activity is controlled by secretion. *FEBS Lett.* **113**, 196–199.

Gerrard, J.M., White, J.G. and Rao G.H.R. (1974). Effects of the ionophore A23187 on the blood platelets. II. Influence on ultrastructure. *J. Pathol.* **77**, 151–166.

Gerrard, J.M., Peterson, D.A. and White, J.G. (1981). Calcium mobilisation. In Gordon, J.L. (ed.) *Platelets in Biology and Pathology 2*. Oxford, Elsevier/North Holland, pp. 407–436.

Gerrard, J.M., White, J.G. and Peterson, D.A. (1978). The platelet dense tubular system: its relationship to prostaglandin synthesis and calcium flux. *Thromb. Haemost.* **40**, 224–231.

Ginsberg, M.H., Painter, R.G., Birdwell, C. et al (1979). The detection, immunofluorescent localization and thrombin-induced release of human platelet-associated fibronectin antigen. *J. Supramol. Struct.* **11**, 167–174.

Giugliano, D., Misso, L., Tirelli, A. et al (1982). Platelet aggregation after strict metabolic control using the artificial pancreas. *Diabetologia* **23**, 545.

Glavind, J., Hartmann, S., Clemmesen, J. et al (1952). Studies on the role of lipoperoxides in human pathology. II. The presence of peroxidized lipids in the atherosclerotic aorts. *Acta Pathol. Microbiol. Scand.* **30**, 1–6.

Goehlert, U.G., Ng Ying Kin, N.M.K. and Wolfe, L.S.

(1981). Biosynthesis of prostacyclin in rat cerebral microvessels and the choroid plexus. *J. Neurochem.* **36**, 1192–1201.

Gorman, R.R., Bunting, S. and Miller, Q.V. (1977). Modulation of human platelet adenylate cyclase by prostacyclin (PGX). *Prostaglandins* **13**, 377–388.

Greaves, M. and Preston, F.E. (1982). Plasma 6-keto-prostaglandin $F_{1\alpha}$ fact or fiction? *Thromb. Res.* **26**, 145–157.

Greenberg, J.H. and Jamieson, G.A. (1974). The effects of various lectins on platelet aggregation and release. *Biochim. Biophys. Acta* **345**, 231–242.

Grette, K. (1962). Studies on the mechanism of thrombin catalysed haemostatic reactions in blood platelets. *Acta Physiol. Scand.* **56**, Suppl. 195.

Grotendorst, G.T., Chang, T., Seppa, H.E.J. et al (1982). Platelet derived growth factor is a chemo-attractant for vascular smooth muscle cells. *J. Cell Physiol.* **113**, 261–266.

Gryglewski, R.J., Bunting, S., Moncada, S. et al (1976). Arterial walls are protected against deposition of platelet thrombi by a substance (prostaglandin X) which they make from a prostaglandin endoperoxide. *Prostaglandins* **12**, 685–714.

Gryglewski, R.J., Dembinska-Kiec, A., Zmuda, A. et al (1978). Prostacyclin and thromboxane A_2 biosynthesis capacities of heart, arteries and platelets of various stages of experimental atherosclerosis in rabbits. *Atherosclerosis* **31**, 385–392.

Haerem, J.W. (1972). Platelet aggregates in intramyocardial vessels of patients dying suddenly and unexpectedly of coronary artery disease. *Atherosclerosis* **15**, 199–213.

Halushka, P.V., Lurie, D. and Colwell, J.A. (1977). Increased synthesis of prostaglandin E-like material by platelets from patients with diabetes mellitus. *N. Engl. J. Med.* **297**, 1306–1310.

Halushka, P.V., Mayfield, R., Wohltmann, H.J., et al (1981a). Increased platelet arachidonic acid metabolism in diabetes mellitus. *Diabetes* **30**, Suppl. 2, 44–48.

Halushka, P.V., Roger, R.C., Loadholt, C.B. et al (1981b). Increased platelet thromboxane synthesis in diabetes mellitus. *J. Lab. Clin. Med.* **97**, 87–96.

Hamberg, M. and Samuelsson, B. (1974). Prostaglandin endoperoxides. Novel transformations of arachidonic acid in human platelets. *Proc. Natl. Acad. Sci. USA* **71**, 3400–3404.

Hamberg, M., Svensson, J. and Samuelsson, B. (1974). Prostaglandin endoperoxides. A new concept concerning the mode of action and release of prostaglandins. *Proc. Natl. Acad. Sci. USA* **71**, 3824–3828.

Hamberg, M., Svenson, J. and Samuelsson, B. (1975). Thromboxanes: a new group of biologically active compounds derived from prostaglandin endoperoxides. *Proc. Natl. Acad. USA* **72**, 2994–2998.

Handin, R.I., McDonough, M. and Lesch, M. (1978). Elevation of platelet factor 4 in acute myocardial infarction. Measurement by radioimmunoassay. *J. Lab. Clin. Med.* **9**, 340–349.

Hardisty, R.M., Hutton, R.A., Montgomery, D. et al (1970). Secondary platelet aggregation: a quantitative study. *Br. J. Haematol.* **19**, 307–319.

Harker, L.A. and Ross, R. (1979). Pathogenesis of arterial vascular disease. *Semin. Thromb. Hemost.* **5**, 274–292.

Harland, W.A., Gilbert, J.D., Steel, G. et al (1971). Lipids of human atheroma. Part 5. The occurrence of a new group of polar sterol esters in various stages of human atherosclerosis. *Atherosclerosis* **13**, 239–246.

Harrison, H.E., Reece, A.H. and Johnson, M. (1978). Decreased vascular prostacyclin in experimental diabetes. *Life* **23**, 351–356.

Harrison, H.E., Reece, A.H. and Johnson, M. (1980). Effect of insulin treatment on prostacyclin in experimental diabetes. *Diabetologia* **18**, 65–68.

Haslam, R.J. and McClenaghan, M.D. (1981). Measurement of circulating prostacyclin. *Nature* **292**, 364–366.

Hassall, D.G., Forrest, L.A., Bruckdorfer, R. et al (1983). Influence of plasma lipoproteins on platelet aggregation in a normal male population. *Arteriosclerosis* **3**, 332–338.

Heath, H., Brigden, W.D., Canever, J.V. et al (1971). Platelet adhesion and aggregation in relation to diabetic retinopathy. *Diabetologia* **7**, 308–315.

Hellem, A.J. (1971). Adenosine diphosphate induced platelet adhesiveness in diabetes mellitus with complications. *Acta Med. Scand.* **190**, 291–295.

Higgs, G.A., Moncada, S., Salmon, J.A. et al (1982). The source of prostaglandins and thromboxanes in experimental inflammation. *Br. J. Pharmacol.* **77**, 492.

Higgs, G.A., Moncada, S. and Vane, J.R. (1977). Prostacyclin inhibits the formation of platelet thrombi induced by adenosine diphosphate (ADP) *in vivo. Br. J. Pharmacol.* **61**, 137.

Higgs, E.A., Moncada, S., Vane, J.R. et al (1978). Effect of prostacyclin (PGI_2) on platelet adhesion to rabbit arterial subendothelium. *Prostaglandins* **16**, 17–22.

Higuchi, Y. (1982). Lipid peroxides and α-tocopherol in rat streptozotocin-induced diabetes mellitus. *Acta Med. Okayama.* **36**, 165–175.

Hilsted, J., Madsbad, D., Dalsgaard-Nielsen J. et al (1980). Hypoglycaemia and haemostatic parameters in juvenile-onset diabetes. *Diabet. Care* **3**, 675–678.

Hirsh, P.D., Hillis, L.D., Campbell, W.D. et al (1981).

Release of prostaglandins and thromboxane into the coronary circulation in patients with ischaemic heart disease. *N. Engl. J. Med.* **304**, 685–691.

Hiti-Harper, J., Wohl, H. and Harper, E. (1978). Platelet factor 4: an inhibitor of collagenase. *Science* **199**, 991–992.

Holmsen, H. (1975). Biochemistry of the platelet release reaction. In *Biochemistry and Pharmacology of Platelets. Ciba Foundation Symposium 35,* Amsterdam, Elsevier Scientific Publishing Company Excerpta Medica, North Holland Publishing Company, pp. 175–205.

Holmsen, H. (1977). In Day, H.J., Holsen, H. and Zucker, M.B. (eds), *Platelet Function Testing,* DHEW Publication No (NIH) 78-1087, US Gov. Printing Office, pp. 112–132.

Holmsen, H., Day, H.J. and Stormorken, H. (1969). The blood platelet release reaction. *Scand. J. Haematol.* **8**, Suppl. 1–39.

Holmsen, H. and Weiss, H.J. (1979). Secretable storage pools in platelets. *Ann. Rev. Med.* **30**, 119–134.

Hope, W., Martin, R.J., Chesterman, C.N. et al (1979). Human β-thromboglobulin inhibits PGI_2 production and binds to a specific site in bovine aortic endothelial cells. *Nature* **282**, 210–212.

Hovig, T., Dodds, W.J., Rowsell, H.C. et al (1968). The transformation of haemostatic plugs in normal and factor IX deficiency individuals. *Am. J. Pathol.* **53**, 355–374.

Howard, B.V., Macarak, E.J., Gunson, D. et al (1976). Characterization of the collagen synthesized by endothelial cells in culture. *Proc. Natl. Acad. Sci. USA* **713**, 2361–2364.

Humphrey, J.H. and Jaques, R. (1955). The release of histamine and 5-HT (serotonin) from platelets by antigen: antibody reactions *in vitro. J. Physiol* (Lond.) **128**, 9–27.

Hutton, R.A., Mikhailidis, D., Dormandy, K.M. et al (1979). Platelet aggregation studies during transient hypoglycaemia. *J. Clin. Pathol.* **32**, 434–438.

Ingerman-Wojenski, C.M., Bryan-Smith, H.J. and Silver, M.J. (1982). Difficulty in detecting inhibition of platelet aggregation by the impedance method. *Thromb. Res.* **28**, 427–432.

Jackson, E.K., Goodman, R.P., Fitzgerald, G.A. et al (1982). Assessment of the extent to which exogenous prostaglandin I_2 is converted to 6-keto-prostaglandin E_1 in human subjects. *J. Pharmacol. Exp. Ther.* **221**, 183–187.

Jackson, C.A., Greaves, M., Boulton, A.J.M. et al (1984). Near normal glycaemic control does not correct abnormal platelet reactivity in diabetes mellitus. *Clin. Sci.* **67**, 551–555.

Jaffe, E.A., Minick, C.R., Adelman, B. et al (1976). Synthesis of basement membrane collagen by cultured human endothelial cells. *J. Exp. Med.* **144**, 209–225.

Janka, H.U., Standl, E., Schramm, W. et al (1983). Platelet enzyme activities in diabetes mellitus in relation to endothelial damage. *Diabetes* **32**, Suppl., 47–53.

Jarrett, R.J., Keen, H. and Chakrabarti R. (1982). Diabetes, hyperglycaemia and arterial disease. In Keen, H. and Jarrett, R.J. (eds), *Complications of Diabetes*, 2nd edn, London, Edward Arnold, pp. 179–204.

Johnson, A.R. and Erdos, E.G. (1977). Metabolism of vasoactive peptides by human endothelial cells in culture. *J. Clin. Invest.* **59**, 684–695.

Johnson, M., Harrison, H.E., Raftery, A.T. et al (1979). Vascular prostacyclin may be reduced in diabetes in man. *Lancet* i, 325–326.

Johnson, M., Reece, A.H. and Harrison, H.E. (1980). An imbalance in arachidonic acid metabolism in diabetes. In Samuelsson, B., Ramwell, P.W. and Paoletti, R. (eds), *Advances in Prostaglandin and Thromboxane Research, Vol. 8,* New York, Raven Press, pp. 1283–1286.

Johnson, R.A., Morton, D.R., Kinner, J.H. et al (1976). Chemical structure of prostaglandin X (prostacyclin). *Prostaglandins* **12**, 915–928.

Joist, J.H., Baker, K. and Schoenfeld, G. (1979). Increased *in vivo* and *in vitro* platelet function in type II and type IV hyperlipoproteinaemia. *Thromb. Res.* **15**, 95–108.

Jones, D.B., Carter, R.D., Haitas, B. et al (1983). Low phospholipid arachidonic acid values in diabetic platelets. *Br. Med. J.* **286**, 173–175.

Jones, R.J., Delamothe, A.P., Curtis, L.D. et al (1985). Measurement of platelet aggregation in diabetics using the new electronic platelet aggregometer. *Diabet. Med.* **2**, 105–109.

Juhan, I., Vague, Ph., Buonocore, M. et al (1982). Abnormalities of erythrocyte deformability and platelet aggregation in insulin dependent diabetics corrected by insulin *in vivo* and *in vitro. Lancet* i, 535–537.

Kaplan, J.L. (1981). Platelet granule proteins: localization and secretion. In Gordon, J.L. (ed.), *Platelets in Biology and Pathology,* Amsterdam, Elsevier/North Holland and Biomedical Press, pp. 77–90.

Kaplan, K.L., Broekman, J., Chernoff, A. et al (1979). Platelet alpha granule proteins: studies on release and subcellular localisation. *Blood* **53**, 604–618.

Kaplan, K.L. and Owen, J. (1981). Plasma levels of β-thromboglobulin and platelet factor 4 as indices of platelet activation *in vivo. Blood* **57**, 199–202.

Käser-Glanzmann, R., Jakabova, M., George, J.N. et al (1977). Stimulation of calcium uptake in platelet vesicles by adenosine 3′, 5′ cyclic monophosphate and protein kinase. *Biochim. Biophys. Acta* **466**, 429–440.

Keen, H. and Jarrett, J. (1982). *Complications of Diabetes*, 2nd edn, London, Edward Arnold.

Khosla, P.K., Mahabaleswara, M., Tiwari, H.K. et al (1979). Platelet aggregation and retinal microangiopathy in diabetes and hypertension. *Acta Haematol. (Basel).* **61**, 161–167.

Kinlough-Rathbone, R.L., Reimers, H.J., Mustard, J.F. et al (1976). Sodium arachidonate can induce platelet shape change and aggregation which are independent of the release reaction. *Science* **192**, 1011–1012.

Klaff, L.J., Vinik, A.I., Jackson, W.P.U. et al (1979). Effects of the sulphonylurea drugs gliclazide and glibenclamide on blood glucose control and platelet function. *South Afr. Med.* **56**, 247–250.

Kohner, E.M. and Baudoin, C.E. (1985). Effect of aspirin and aspirin combined with dipyridamole in early diabetic retinopathy. *Diabet. Res. Clin. Pract.* Suppl. 1, S312–313.

Krzywanek, H.M. and Breddin, H. (1981). Platelet aggregation as a risk factor in diabetic subjects. *Horm. Metab. Res.* **11**, Suppl., 11–14.

Kwaan, H.C., Colwell, J.A. and Suwanawela, N. (1972). Disseminated intravascular coagulation in diabetes mellitus, with reference to the role of increased platelet aggregation. *Diabetes* **21**, 108–113.

Lagarde, M., Burtin, M., Berciaud, P. et al (1980). Increase of platelet thromboxane A_2 formation and of its plasmatic half-life in diabetes mellitus. *Thromb. Res.* **19**, 823–830.

Lagarde, M. and Dechavanne, M. (1977). Increase of platelet prostaglandin cyclic endoperoxides in thrombosis. *Lancet* **i**, 88.

Lagarde, M., Dechavanne, M., Thouverez, J.-P. et al (1975). Effect of gliclazide, a new anti-diabetic agent, on the platelet release reaction role of adenylate cyclase. *Thromb. Res.* **6**, 345–355.

Lands, W.E.M. (1979). The biosynthesis and metabolism of prostaglandins. *Ann. Rev. Physiol.* **41**, 633–652.

Larrue, J., Rigaud, M., Daret, D. et al (1980). Prostacyclin production by cultured smooth muscle cells from atherosclerotic rabbit aorta. *Nature* **285**, 480–482.

Lasche, E.M. and Larson, R.E. (1982). Interaction of insulin and prostacyclin production in the rat. *Diabetes* **31**, 454–458.

Lewy, R.I., Smith, J.B., Silver, M.J. et al (1979). Detection of thromboxane B_2 in peripheral blood of patients with Prinzmetal's angina. *Prostaglandins* **2**, 243–248.

Lieberman, G.E., Lewis, P. and Peters, T.J. (1977). A membrane-bound enzyme in rabbit aorta capable of inhibiting adenosine diphosphate-induced platelet aggregation. *Lancet* **ii**, 330–332.

Lindahl, S.P. and Hook, M. (1978). Glycosaminoglycans and their binding to biological macromolecules. *Ann. Rev. Biochem.* **47**, 385–417.

Lollar, P. and Owen, W.G. (1980). Clearance of thrombin from the circulation by high affinity binding sites on endothelium: possible role in the inactivation of thrombin by antithrombin III. *Circulation* **62**, Suppl. III, 278.

Lorenz, R., Spengler, U., Fischer, S. et al (1983). Platelet function, thromboxane formation and blood pressure control during supplementation of the Western diet with cod liver oil. *Circulation* **67** 504–511.

Loskutoff, D.J. and Edgington, T.S. (1977). Synthesis of a fibrinolytic activator and inhibitor by endothelial cells. *Proc. Natl. Acad. Sci. USA* **74**, 3903–3907.

Lucas, R.C. Detwiler, T.C. and Stracher, A. (1976). The identification and isolation of a high molecular weight (270,000 dalton) actin-binding protein from human platelets. *J. Cell Biol.* **70**, 259a.

Ludlam, C.A. (1979). Evidence for the platelet specificity of β-thromboglobin and studies on its concentration in healthy individuals. *Br. J. Haematol.* **41**, 271–278.

Ludlam, C.A., Bolton, A.E., Moore, S. et al (1975). New rapid method for diagnosis of deep venous thrombosis. *Lancet* **ii**, 259–260.

Lundbaek, K. (1973). Diabetic angiopathy. *Acta Diabetol.* **10**, 183–207.

McDonald, J.W., Dupre, J., Rodger, N.W. et al (1982). Comparison platelet thromboxane synthesis in diabetic patients on conventional insulin therapy and continuous insulin infusions. *Thromb. Res.* **28**, 705–712.

MacIntyre, D.E. (1979). Modulation of platelet function by prostaglandins: characterization of platelet receptors for stimulatory prostaglandins and the role of arachidonate metabolites in platelet degranulation responses. *Haemostasis* **8**, 274–293.

MacIntyre, D.E. (1981). Platelet prostaglandin receptors. In Gordon, J.L. (ed.), *Platelets in Biology and Pathology - 2*, Amsterdam, Elsevier/North Holland Press, pp. 211–247.

McManus, L.M., Morley, C.A., Levine, S.P. et al (1979). Platelet activating factor (PAF) induced release of platelet factor 4 (PF_4) *in vitro* and during IgE anaphylaxis in the rabbit. *J. Immunol.* **123**, 2835–2841.

MacMillan, D.C. (1966). Secondary clumping effect in human citrated platelet-rich plasma produced by adenosine diphosphate and adrenaline. *Nature* **211**, 140–144.

Majno, G. and Joris, I. (1978). Endothelium 1977: a review. *Adv. Exp. Med. Biol.* **104**, 169–225.

Malmsten, C., Granstrom, E. and Samuelsson, B. (1976). Cyclic AMP inhibits synthesis of prostaglandin endoperoxide (PGG_2) in human platelets. *Biochem. Biophys. Res. Commun.* **68**, 569–576.

Massini, P. and Luscher, E.F. (1974). Some effects of ionophores for divalent cations on blood platelets—a comparison with the effects of thrombin. *Biochim. Biophys. Acta* **372**, 109–121.

Mathews, J.H., O'Connor, J.F., Hearnshaw, J.R. et al (1979). β-Thromboglobulin and glycosylated haemoglobin in diabetes mellitus. *Scand. J. Haematol.* **23**, 421–426.

Mayne, E.E., Bridges, J.M. and Weaver, J.A. (1970). Platelet adhesiveness, plasma fibrinogen and factor VIII levels in diabetes mellitus. *Diabetologia* **6**, 436–440.

Miale, J.B. and Kent, J.W. (1975). Prothrombin comple protein as cofactor in aggregation. I: Inhibition of aggregation by antiserum. *Blood* **45**, 97–106.

Mickel, H.S. and Horbar, J. (1974). The effect of peroxidized arachidonic acid upon human platelet aggregation. *Lipids* **9**, 68–71.

Miettinen, T.A. (1974). Hyperlipoproteinaemia—relation to platelet lipids, platelet function and tendency to thrombosis. *Thromb. Res.* **4**, Suppl., 41–47.

Miller, O.V. and Gorman, R.R. (1979). Evidence for distinct PGI_2 and PGD_2 receptors in human platelets. *J. Pharmacol. Exp. Ther.* **210**, 134–140.

Mills, D.C.B. (1981). The basic biochemistry of the platelet. In Bloom, A.L. and Thomas, D.P. (eds.), *Haemostasis and Thrombosis*, Churchill Livingstone, Edinburgh. pp. 50–60.

Mills, D.C.B., Robb, I.A. and Roberts, G.C.K. (1968). The release of nucleotides 5-hydroxytryptamine and enzymes from human blood platelets during aggregation. *J. Physiol. (Lond.)* **195**, 715–729.

Minkes, M., Stanford, M., Chi, M. et al (1977). Cyclic adenosine 3′, 5′-monophosphate inhibits the availability of arachidonate to prostaglandin synthetase in human platelet suspensions. *J. Clin. Invest.* **59**, 449–454.

Mitchell, J.R.A. and Sharp, A.A. (1964). Platelet clumping in vitro. *Br. J. Haematol.* **10**, 78–93.

Miyamoto, T., Yamamoto, S. and Hayaishi, O. (1974). Prostaglandin synthetase system-resolution into oxygenase and isomerase components. *Proc. Natl. Acad. Sci. USA* **71**, 3645–3648.

Moncada, S., Gryglewski, R.J., Bunting, S. et al (1976a). An enzyme isolated from arteries transforms prostaglandin endoperoxides to an unstable substance that inhibits platelet aggregation. *Nature* **263**, 663–665.

Moncada, S., Gryglewski, R.J., Bunting, S. et al (1976b). A lipid peroxide inhibits the enzyme in blood vessel microsomes that generates from prostaglandin endoperoxides the substance (prostaglandin X) which prevents platelet aggregation. *Prostaglandins* **12**, 715–733.

Moncada, S., Herman, A.G., Higgs, E.A. et al (1977). Differential formation of prostacyclin (PGX or PGI_2) by layers of the arterial wall. An explanation for the anti-thrombotic properties of vascular endothelium. *Thromb. Res.* **11**, 323–344.

Moncada, S. and Vane, J.R. (1978). Unstable metabolites of arachidonic acid and their role in haemostasis and thrombosis. *Br. Med. Bull.* **34**, 129–135.

Moncada, S. and Vane, J.R. (1979). Pharmacology and endogenous roles of prostaglandin endoperoxides, thromboxane A_2 and prostacyclin. *Pharmacol. Rev.* **30**, 293–331.

Monnier, L.H., Lachkar, H., Richard, J.L. et al (1984). Plasma β-thromboglobulin in response to insulin-induced hypoglycaemia in type I diabetic patients. *Diabetes* **33**, 907–909.

Moore, S., Pepper, D.S. and Cash, J.D. (1975). The isolation and characterization of platelet specific β-globulin (β-thromboglobulin) and the detection of anti-urokinase and anti-plasmin released from thrombin-aggregated washed human platelets. *Biochim. Biophys. Acta* **379**, 360–369.

Mueller-Eckhardt, Ch. and Luscher, E.F. (1968). Immune reactions of human blood platelets. I. A comparative study of the effects on platelets of heterologous anti-platelet anti-serum antigen–antibody complexes, aggregated gammaglobulin and thrombin. *Throm. Diath. Haemorrh.* **20**, 155–167.

Murphy, E.A., Rowsell, H.C. Downie, H.G. et al (1962). Encrustation and atherosclerosis. The analogy between early *in vivo* lesions and deposits which occur in extracorporeal circulations. *Can. Med. Assoc. J.* **87**, 259–274.

Mustard, J.F., Packham, M.A. Kinlough-Rathbone, R.L. et al (1978). Fibrinogen and ADP induced platelet aggregation. *Blood* **52**, 453–466.

Mustard, J.F., Packham, M.A. and Kinlough-Rathbone, R.L. (1983). Platelets and atherosclerosis. In Miller, N.E. (ed.) *Atherosclerosis: Mechanisms and Approaches to Therapy*, New York, Raven Press, pp. 29–43.

Musial, J., Niewiarowski, S., Edmunds, L.H.Jr. et al (1980). *In vivo* release and turnover of secreted platelet antiheparin proteins in rhesus monkey (Macaca mulatta). *Blood* **56**, 596–602.

Needleman, P., Moncada, S., Bunting, S. et al (1976). Identification of an enzyme in platelet microsomes which generates thromboxane A_2 from prostaglandin endoperoxides. *Nature* **261**, 558–560.

Niewiarowski, S. (1977). Proteins secreted by the platelets. *Thromb. Haemost.* **38**, 924–938.

Niewiarowski, S., Budzynski, A.Z. and Lipinski, B.

(1971). Significance of the intact polypeptide chains of human fibrinogen in ADP-induced platelet aggregation. *Blood* **49**, 635–644.

Niewiarowski, S. and Paul D. (1981). Platelet granule proteins with mitogenic and antiheparin activity. In Gordon, J.L. (ed.), *Platelets in Biology and Pathology 2*, Amsterdam, Elsevier/North Holland and Biomedical Press, pp. 92–106.

Niewiarowski, S., Poplawski, A., Lipinski, B. et al (1969). The release of platelet factor 4 during platelet aggregation and the possible significance of this reaction in haemostasis. *Experientia* **24**, 343–344.

Niewiarowski, S., Rucinski, B., James, P. et at (1979). Platelet antiheparin proteins and antithrombin III interact with different binding sites on heparin molecule. *FEBS Lett.* **102**, 75–78.

Nishigaki, I., Hagihara, M., Tsunekawa, H. et al (1981). Lipid peroxide levels in serum lipoprotein fractions of diabetic patients. *Biochem. Med.* **25**, 373–378.

Nordoy, A. and Rodset, J.M. (1971). Platelet function and platelet phospholipids in patients with hyperbetalipoproteinaemia. *Acta. Med. Scand.* **189**, 385–389.

Nugteren, D.H. (1975). Arachidonate lipoxygenase in blood platelets. *Biochim. Biophys. Acta* **380**, 299–307.

Nugteren, D.H. and Hazelhof, E. (1973). Isolation and properties of intermediates in prostaglandin biosynthesis. *Biochim. Biophys. Acta* **380**, 299–307.

Nurden, A.T. and Caen, J.P. (1974). An abnormal platelet glycoprotein pattern in three cases of Glanzmann's thrombasthenia. *Br. J. Haematol.* **28**, 253–260.

Nurden, A.T. and Caen, J.P. (1975). Specific roles for platelet surface glycoproteins in platelet function. *Nature* **255**, 720–722.

O'Malley, B.C., Ward, J.D., Timperly, W.R. et al (1975). Platelet abnormalities in diabetic peripheral neuropathy. *Lancet* **ii**, 1274–1276.

Onodera, H., Hirata, T., Sugawara, H. et al (1981). Platelet sensitivity to adenosine diphosphate and to prostacyclin in diabetic patients. *Tohoku J. Exp. Med.* **137**, 423–428.

Owen, A.J., Geyer, R.P. and Antoniades, H.N. (1982). Human platelet-derived growth factor stimulates amino acid transport and protein synthesis by human diploid fibroblasts in plasma-free medium. *Proc. Natl Acad. Sci. USA* **79**, 3203–3207.

Packham, M.A. (1976). Stages in the interaction of platelets with collagen. *Thromb. Haemost.* **36**, 269–272.

Paisey, R., Elkeles, R.S., Hambley, J. et al (1978). The effect of chlorpropamide and insulin on serum lipids, lipoproteins and fractional triglyceride removal. *Diabetologia* **15**, 81–85.

Patel, M.K., Evans, C.E. and McEvoy, F.A. (1983). 6-Keto-prostaglandin $F_{1\alpha}$ production in endothelial-cell cultures in response to normal and diabetic human serum. *Biosci. Rep.* **3**, 53–60.

Paton, R.C. (1981). Haemostatic changes in diabetic coma. *Diabetologia* **21**, 172–177.

Paton, R.C., Guillot, R., Passa, P. et al (1982a). Prostacyclin production by human endothelial cells cultured in diabetic serum. *Diabet. Metab.* (1982). **8**: 323–328.

Paton, R.C., Kernoff, P.B.A., Wales, J.K. et al (1982b). Effects of diet and gliclazide on the haemostatic system of non-insulin-dependent diabetics. *Br. Med. J.* **283**, 1018–1020.

Paulsen, E.P., McChung, N.M. and Sabio, H. (1981). Some characteristics of spontaneous platelet aggregation in young insulin-dependent diabetic subjects. *Horm. Metab. Res.* **ii**, Suppl., 15–21.

Peerschke, E.I., Zucker, M.B., Grant, R.A. et al (1980). Correlation between fibrinogen binding to human platelets and platelet aggregability. *Blood* **55**, 841–847.

Petersen, H.D. and Gormsen, J. (1978). Platelet aggregation in diabetes mellitus. *Acta Med. Scand.* **203**, 125–130.

Peterson, C.M., Jones, R.L., Koenig, R.J. et al (1977). Reversible haematologic sequeles of diabetes mellitus. *Ann. Intern. Med.* **86**, 425–429.

Phillips, D.R. and Agin, P.P. (1977). Platelet membrane defects in Glanzmann's thrombasthenia. Evidence for decreased amounts of two major glucoproteins. *J. Clin. Invest.* **60**, 535–545.

Piper, P.J. and Vane, J.R. (1969). Release of additional factors in anaphylaxis and its antagonism by anti-inflammatory drugs. *Nature* **223**, 29–35.

Poari, O., Civardi, E., Megha, S. et al (1979). Antiplatelet effects of long-term treatment with gliclazide in diabetic patients. *Thromb. Res.* **16**, 191–203.

Pollard, T.D. (1975). Functional implications of the biochemical and structural properties of cytoplasmic contractile proteins. In Inoise, S. and Stephens, R.D. (eds.), *Molecules and Cell Movement*, Raven Press, New York, pp. 259–274.

Preston, F.E., Ward, J.D., Marcola, B.H. et al (1978). Elevated β-thromboglobulin levels and circulating platelet aggregates in diabetic microangiopathy. *Lancet* **i**, 238–240.

Quick, A.J. (1966). Salicylates and bleeding: the aspirin tolerance test. *Am. J. Med. Sci.* **252**, 265–269.

Quilley, C.P., McGiff, J.C., Lee, W.H. et al (1980). 6-Keto-PGE_1: a possible metabolite of prostacyclin having platelet antiaggregatory effects. *Hypertension* **2**, 524–528.

Rak, K., Beck, P., Udvardy, M. et al (1983). Plasma levels of beta-thromboglobulin and factor VIII-related antigen in diabetic children and adults. *Thromb. Res.* **29**, 155–162.

Richardson, P.D., Galetti, P. and Born, G.V.R. (1976). Regional administration of drugs to control thombosis in artificial organs. *Trans. Am. Soc. Artif. Intern. Organs* **22**, 22–29.

Rittenhouse-Simmons, D. (1979). Production of diglyceride from phosphatidylinositol in activated human platelets. *J. Clin. Invest.* **63**, 580–587.

Rizza, R.A., Cryer, P.E. and Gerich, J.E. (1979). Role of glucagon, catecholamines and growth hormone in human glucose counterregulation. *J. Clin. Invest.* **64**, 62–71.

Robertson, R.M., Robertson, D., Roberts, J. et al (1981). Thromboxane A_2 in vasotonic angina pectoris: evidence from direct measurements and inhibitor trials. *N. Engl. J. Med.* **304**, 998–1003.

Robertson, W.B. and Strong, J.P. (1968). Atherosclerosis in persons with hypertension and diabetes mellitus. *Lab. Invest.* **18**, 538–551.

Rogers, S.P. and Larkins, R.G. (1981). Production of 6-oxo-prostaglandin $F_{1\alpha}$ by rat aorta influence of diabetes, insulin treatment and caloric deprivation. *Diabetes* **30**, 935–939.

Rohrer, T.F., Pfister, B., Weber, C. et al (1978). Validity of the Wu-Hoak method for the quantitative determination of platelet aggregation *in vivo*. *Blut* **36**, 15–20.

Roos, H. and Pfleger, K. (1972). Kinetics of adenosine uptake by erythrocytes and the influence of dipyridamole. *Mol. Pharmacol.* **8**, 417–425.

Rosove, M.H., Frank, H.J.L. and Harwig, S.S.L. (1984). Plasma β-thromboglobulins, platelet factor 4, fibrinopeptide A and other haemostatic functions during improved short-term glycaemic control in diabetes mellitus. *Diabet. Care* **7**, 174–179.

Ross, R. and Glomset, J. (1976). The pathogenesis of atherosclerosis. *N. Engl. J. Med.* **295**, 369–377.

Ross, R., Glomset, J., Kariya, B. et al (1974). A platelet-dependent serum factor that stimulates the proliferation of arterial smooth muscle cells *in vitro*. *Proc. Natl Acad. Sci. USA* **71**, 1207–1210.

Ross, R. and Vogel, A. (1978). The platelet-derived growth factor. *Cell* **14**, 203–210.

Roth, J., Prout, T.E., Goldfine, I.D. et al (1971). Sulphonylureas, mechanisms and actions. *Ann. Intern. Med.* **75**, 607–621.

Sagel, J., Colwell, J.A., Crook, L. et al (1975). Increased platelet aggregation in early diabetes mellitus. *Ann. Intern. Med.* **82**, 733–738.

Samuelsson, B. (1977). The role of prostaglandin endoperoxides and thromboxanes in human platelets. In Silver, M.J., Smith, J.B. and Kocsis, J.J. (eds.), *Prostaglandins in Haematology*, Spectrum Publications, New York, pp. 1–10.

Salmon, J.A., Smith, D.R., Flower, R.J. et al (1978).

Further studies on the enzymatic conversion of prostaglandin endoperoxide into prostacyclin by porcine aorta microsomes. *Biochim. Biophys. Acta* **523**, 250–262.

Sawyer, P.N. and Srinivasan, S. (1973). The role of surface phenomena in intravascular thrombosis. *Biblthcs Anat No. 12.* Basel, Karger, pp. 106–119.

Schick, P.K. (1979). The role of platelet membrane lipids in platelet haemostatic activities. *Semin. Hematol.* **16**, 221–223.

Schollmeyer, J.V., Rao, G.H.R. and White, J.G. (1978). An actin-binding protein in human platelets: interactions with α-actinin on gelation of actin and the influence of cytochalasin B. *Am. J. Pathol.* **93**, 433–446.

Schwartz, S.M., Gajdusek, C.M., Reidy, M.A. et al (1980). Maintenance of integrity in aortic endothelium. *Fed. Proc.* **39**, 2618–2625.

Seppä, H., Grotendorst, G., Seppä, S. et al (1982). Platelet-derived growth factor is chemotatic for fibroblasts. *J. Cell Biol.* **92**, 584–588.

Shattil, S.J., Anaya-Galindo, R., Bennett, J. et al (1975). Platelet hypersensitivity induced by cholesterol incorporation. *J. Clin. Invest.* **55**, 636–643.

Shattil, S.J. and Bennett, J.S. (1981). Platelets and their membranes in haemostasis: physiology and pathophysiology. *Ann. Intern. Med.* **94**, 108–118.

Shattil, S.J., Bennett, J.S., Colman, R.W. et al (1977). Abnormality of cholesterol-phospholipid composition in platelets and low density lipoproteins of human hyperbetalipoproteinaemia. *J. Lab. Clin. Med.* **89**, 341–353.

Shattil, S.J. and Cooper, R.A. (1976). Membrane microviscosity and human platelet function. *Biochemistry* **15**, 4832–4837.

Shaw, S., Pegrum, G.D., Wolff, S. et al (1967). Platelet adhesiveness in diabetes mellitus. *J. Clin. Pathol.* **20**, 845–847.

Shepherd, G.L., Lewis, P.J., Blair, I.A. et al (1983). Epoprostenol (prostacyclin, PGI_2) binding and activation of adenylate cyclase in platelets of diabetic and control subjects. *Br. J. Clin. Pharmacol.* **15**, 77–81.

Siegel, M.I., McConnel, R.T., Abrahams, S.L. et al (1979). Regulation of arachidonate metabolism via lipoxygenase and cyclo-oxygenase by 12-HPETE, the product of human platelet lipoxygenase. *Biochem. Biophys. Res. Commun.* **89**, 1273–1280.

Siess, W., Roth, P., Scherer, B., Kurzman, I., Bohlig, B. and Weber, P.C. (1980). Platelet membrane fatty acids, platelet aggregation and thromboxane formation during a mackeral diet. *Lancet* i, 441–444.

Silberbauer, K., Clopath, P., Sinzinger, H. et al (1980). Effect of experimentally induced diabetes on swine vascular prostacyclin (PGI_2) synthesis. *Artery* **8**, 30–36.

Silberbauer, K., Schernthaner, G., Sinzinger, H. et al (1979). Decreased vascular prostacyclin in juvenile-onset diabetes. *N. Engl. J. Med.* **300**, 366–367.

Silberbauer, K., Schernthaner, G., Sinzinger, H. et al (1981). Platelet aggregation and reversible platelet aggregates in type 1 diabetes staged by retinal fluorescein angiography. *Atherosclerosis* **4**, 81–90.

Simionescu, N., Simionescu, M. and Palade, G.E. (1976). Structural–functional correlates in the transendothelial change of water-soluble macromolecules. *Thromb. Res.* **8**, Suppl. II, 257–269.

Simpson, R.W., Mann, J.I., Hockaday, T.D.R. et al (1979). Lipid abnormalities in untreated maturity onset diabetics and the effect of treatment. *Diabetologia* **16**, 101–106.

Sinha, A.K., Shattil, S.J. and Colman, R.W. (1977). Cyclic AMP metabolism in cholesterol-rich platelets. *J. Biol. Chem.* **252**, 3310–3314.

Sinzinger, H., Feigl, W. and Silberbauer, K. (1979). Prostacyclin generation in atherosclerotic arteries. *Lancet* ii, 469.

Sixma, J.J. and Wester, J. (1977). The haemostatic plug. *Semin. Hematol.* **14**, 265–299.

Skaer, R.J. (1981). Platelet degranulation. In Gordon, J.L. (ed.), *Platelet Biology and Pathology 2*, Amsterdam, Elsevier/North Holland Biomedical Press, pp. 323–348.

Smith, E.B., Staples, E.M., Dietz, H.S. et al (1979). Role of endothelium in sequestration of lipoprotein and fibrinogen in aortic lesions, thrombi and graft pseudointimas. *Lancet* ii, 812–816.

Smith, J.B. and Willis, A.L. (1971). Aspirin selectively inhibits prostaglandin production in human platelets. *Nature (New Biol.)* **231**, 237–239.

Steer, M.L., MacIntyre, D.E., Levine, L. et al (1980). Is prostacyclin a physiologically important circulating anti-platelet agent. *Nature* **283**, 194–195.

Stewart, M., Doublas, J.T., Lowe, G.D.O. et al (1983). Plasma betathromboglobulin and fibrinopeptide A in transient cerebal ischaemia: raised plasma beta-thromboglobulin predicts high risk patients. *Thromb. Haemost.* **50**, 373.

Stout, R.W. (1981). Blood glucose and atherosclerosis. *Arteriosclerosis* **1**, 227–335.

Strandness, D.E.Jr, Priest, R.E. and Gibbons, E.E. (1964). Combined clinical and pathological study of diabetic and non-diabetic peripheral arterial disease. *Diabetes* **13**, 366–372.

Stuart, M.J., Elrad, H., Graeber, J.E. et al (1979). Increased synthesis of prostaglandin endoperoxides and platelet hyperfunction in infants of mothers with diabetes mellitus. *J. Lab. Clin. Med.* **94**, 12–17.

Subbiah, M.T.R. and Deitemeyer, D. (1980). Altered synthesis of prostaglandins in platelets and aorta from spontaneously diabetic Wistar rats. *Biochem. Med.* **23**, 231–235.

Szczeklik, A., Gryglewski, R.J., Musial, J. et al (1978). Thromboxane generation and platelet aggregation in survivors of myocardial infarction. *Thromb. Diath. Haemorrh.* **40**, 66–74.

Szirtes, M. (1970). Platelet aggregation in diabetes mellitus. *Adv. Cardiol.* **4**, 179–186.

Tateson, J.E., Moncada, S. and Vane, J.R. (1977). Effects of prostacyclin (PGX) on cyclic AMP concentrations in human platelets. *Prostaglandins* **13**, 389–399.

Taylor, K., Glagov, S., Lamberti, J. et al (1978). Surface configuration of early atheromatous lesions in controlled-pressure perfusion-fixed monkey aortas. *Scan. Electron Microsc.* **2**, 449–457.

Thorgeirsson, G. and Gustafson, A. (1981). Effect of vascular endothelium-pathobiologic significance. *Am. J. Pathol.* **93**, 803–848.

Thorngren, M. and Gustafson, A. (1981). Effect of eleven week increase in dietary eicosapentaenoic acid on bleeding time, lipids and platelet aggregation. *Lancet* ii, 1190–1193.

Tremoli, E., Maderna, P., Sirtori, M. et al (1979). Platelet aggregation and malonaldehyde formation in type IIa hypercholesterolaemic patients. *Haemostasis* **8**, 47–53.

Tsuboi, T., Fujitani, B., Maeda, J. et al (1981). Effect of gliclazide on prostaglandin and thromboxane synthesis in guinea pig platelets. *Thromb. Res.* **21**, 103–110.

Ubatuba, F.B., Moncada, S. and Vane, J.R. (1979). The effect of prostacyclin (PGI$_2$) on platelet behaviour, thrombus formation *in vivo* and bleeding time. *Thromb. Diath. Haemorrh.* **41**, 425–434.

Valdorf-Hansen, F. (1967). Thrombocytes and coagulability in diabetics. *Dan. Med. Bull* **14**, 244–248.

van Dorp, D.A., Buytenhek, M., Hazelhof, E.C. et al (1978). Isolation and properties of enzymes involved in prostaglandin biosynthesis. *Acta Biol. Med. Ger.* **37**, 691–699.

Vargaftig, B.B., Chignard, M. and Beneviste, J. (1981). Present concepts of the mechanism of platelet aggregation. *Biochem. Pharmacol.* **30**, 263–271.

Voisin, P.J., Rouselle, D., Streiff, F. et al (1983). Reduction of beta-thromboglobulin levels in diabetics controlled by artificial pancreas. *Metabolism* **32**, 138–141.

Walsh, P.N. (1981). Platelets and coagulation proteins. *Fed. Proc.* **40**, 2086–2091.

Weksler, B.B., Marcus, A.J. and Jaffe, E.A. (1977). Synthesis of prostaglandin I$_2$ (prostacyclin) by cultured human and bovine endothelial cells. *Proc. Natl Acad. Sci. USA* **74**, 3922–3926.

Wester, J., Sixma, J.J., Geuze, J.J. et al (1979). Morphology of the haemostatic plug in human skin wounds. *Lab. Invest.* **41**, 182–192.

White, J.G. (1969). The submembrane filaments of

blood platelets. *Am. J. Pathol.* **56**, 267–277.

White, J.G. (1971). Platelet morphology. In Johnson, J.A. (ed.), *The Circulating Platelet*, London, Academic Press, pp. 45–121.

White, J.G. (1972). Interaction of membrane systems in blood platelets. *Am. J. Pathol.* **66**, 295–312.

White, J.G. (1973). Identification of platelet secretion in the electron microscope. *Ser. Haematol.* **6**, 429–459.

White, J.G. (1974). Electron microscopic studies of platelet secretion. *Prog. Haemost. Thromb.* **2**, 49–98.

White, J.G., Clawson, C.C. and Gerrard, J.M. (1981). Platelet ultrastructure. In Bloom, A.L. and Thomas, D.O. (eds) *Haemostasis and Thombosis*, Edinburgh, Churchill Livingstone, pp. 22–49.

Whittle, B.J.R. and Moncada, S. (1983). Pharmacological interactions between prostacyclin and thromboxanes. *Br. Med. Bull.* **39**, 232–238.

Willis, A.L. and Kuhn, D.C. (1973). New potential mediator of arterial thrombosis whose biosynthesis is inhibited by aspirin. *Prostaglandins* **4**, 127–130.

Wilner, G.D., Nossel, H.L. and LeRoy, E.D. (1969). Aggregation of platelets by collagen. *J. Clin. Invest.* **47**, 2616–2621.

Winocour, P.D., Lopes-Virella, M., Laimins, M. et al (1983). Time course of changes in *in vitro* platelet function and plasma von Willebrand factor activity (VIIIR:WF) and factor VIII-related antigen (VIIIR:Ag) in the diabetic rat. *J. Lab. Clin. Med.* **102**, 795–804.

Wong, P.Y-K., Lee, W.H., Chao, P.H-W. et al (1980). Metabolism of prostacyclin by 9-hydroxy prostaglandin dehydrogenase in human platelets. Formation of a potent inhibitor of platelet aggregation and

enzyme purification. *J. Biol. Chem.* **255**, 9021–9024.

Woolf, N. (1983). Pathology of atherosclerosis. In Miller, N.E. (ed.), *Atherosclerosis: Mechanisms and Approaches to Therapy*, New York, Raven Press, pp. 1–27.

Wörner, P. and Patscheke, H. (1980). Hyperactivity by an enhancement of the arachidonate pathway of platelets treated with cholesterol-rich phospholipid dispersions. *Thromb. Res.* **18**, 439–451.

Wu, K.K. and Hoak, J.C. (1974). A new method for the quantitative detection of platelet aggregates in patients with arterial insufficiency. *Lancet* **ii**, 924–926.

Zahavi, J., Betteridge, D.J., Jones, N.A.G. et al (1981). Enhanced *in vivo* platelet release reaction and prostaglandin synthesis in patients with hyperlipidaemia. *Am. J. Med.* **70**, 59–64.

Zahavi, J., Jones, N.A.G., Leyton, J. et al (1980). Enhanced *in vivo* platelet release reaction in old healthy individuals. *Thromb. Res.* **17**, 329–336.

Ziboh, V.A., Maruta, H., Lords, J. et al (1979). Increased biosynthesis of thromboxane A_2 by diabetic platelets. *Eur. J. Clin. Invest.* **9**, 223–228.

Zucker, M.B. and Borelli, J. (1962). Platelet clumping produced by connective tissue suspensions and by collagen. *Proc. Soc. Exp. Biol. Med.* **109**, 779–781.

Zucker, M.B., Mosesson, M.W., Broekman, M.J. et al (1979). Release of platelet fibronectin (cold insoluble globulin) from alpha granules induced by thrombin or collagen: lack of requirement for plasma fibronectin in ADP induced platelet aggregation. *Blood* **54**, 8–12.

Zucker-Franklin, D. (1970). The submembraneous fibrils of human platelets. *J. Cell. Biol.* **47**, 293–299.

Chapter Six

Managing Diabetes

K.G. Taylor

Dr Ken Taylor qualified and spent his early training years in London. His MD research project at St Bartholomew's Hospital concerned lipid metabolism in relation to diabetes. In 1978 he took up a Senior Registrar post in Diabetes at the General Hospital, Birmingham, and in 1981 his present post as Consultant Physician at Dudley Road Hospital, Birmingham. His special interests include factors contributing to the development of atheroma and its complications and prevention by ensuring that patients benefit fully from the practical application of current knowledge and developments.

During Myocardial Infarction

From the earlier chapters it is apparent that myocardial infarction is an all-too-frequent occurrence in diabetic patients, whether they are insulin-dependent or not. Mortality is 33–38 per cent as opposed to 17–18 per cent in the non-diabetic population (Partamian et al, 1965; Czyzk et al, 1980; Gwilt et al, 1984). Possible reasons for this 2-fold difference are as follows. Myocardial infarction may lead to increased secretion of counter-regulatory hormones, catecholamines and cortisol which antagonise the actions of insulin and cause a deterioration in the metabolic environment. Elevation of blood glucose, ketone bodies and free fatty acids in particular may be deleterious to the injured area of myocardium and predispose to arrhythmias (Oliver et al, 1968), impaired contractility or larger infarcts (Kjekshus and Mjøs, 1972; Liedtke et al, 1978; Vik-Mo & Mjøs, 1981)

compared to non-diabetics, predisposing to cardiogenic shock or left ventricular failure. Diabetic patients may have a damaged myocardium due to extensive atheroma and/or small-vessel cardiomyopathy before infarction (Hamby et al, 1974; Regan et al, 1977; Factor et al, 1980), which would make them more likely to develop cardiogenic shock or heart failure.

A study to determine if excellent metabolic control reduced the mortality from myocardial infarction in patients with diabetes was disappointingly negative (Gwilt et al, 1984), but a similar study on a smaller number of patients in Scotland showed considerable benefit (Clark et al, 1985) indicating the need for further investigation. Pre-existing disease of the coronary macro-circulation and perhaps microcirculation may be the most important factors affecting mortality from acute myocardial infarction in diabetic patients.

Although there may not be any benefit on

mortality from very good diabetic control immediately following myocardial infarction, it is clearly undesirable to have uncontrolled diabetes at this time. An interesting feature that has emerged recently is the number of patients who are newly diagnosed as diabetic at the time of their myocardial infarction (Oswald et al, 1984). This study suggested an overall prevalence of undiagnosed diabetes of 5.3 per cent in patients presenting with acute infarction. It used to be thought that this was temporary diabetes resulting from the stress of infarction, but present data suggest that these patients have undiagnosed diabetes before infarction (Husband et al, 1983; Oswald et al, 1984).

Clearly those looking after patients following infarction need to be aware that a significant number will be known diabetics and some will have undiagnosed diabetes, and they will all tend to have a higher mortality than non-diabetics. Myocardial infarction will tend to cause a deterioration in the diabetes. It goes without saying that testing of the urine for glucose and ketones should be mandatory for all patients admitted with infarction and this should be continually charted for those found to be diabetic. Ketonuria is an important indicator that diabetes is inadequately controlled. While urine testing remains the single most useful screening test for diabetes and the adequacy of its management, blood testing in addition provides definitive information and avoids the pitfall of a high renal threshold not uncommon in older patients, or the problem of not having a urine specimen immediately available. A reasonable course is to measure the blood glucose of all patients when they present with infarction. For known diabetics the blood glucose can be rechecked four-hourly for at least the first 48 hours. An alternative to blood testing by the laboratory is the use of a test strip in conjunction with a reflectance meter. This is standard now in many coronary care units and is reliable provided staff are competent with the technique. If the blood glucose is above 20 mmol/l a sample should be sent to the laboratory for a definitive result.

Although infarction can be expected to disturb diabetes it does not invariably do so. For some patients observation with little change in regime may be all that is necessary. The diet following infarction will obviously be quite light. Non-insulin-dependent patients may be receiving diet alone, or diet and oral hypoglycaemic agents. Undoubtedly metformin therapy should be discontinued as this drug can predispose to lactic acidosis if tissue hypoxia occurs (Bergman et al, 1978; Luft et al, 1978; Nattrass & Alberti, 1978). This is more likely following infarction when cardiac output may be reduced and therefore tissue perfusion impaired. If patients are receiving sulphonylureas at the time of admission there is no contraindication to their continuation, although one should be wary of the very long-acting chlorpropamide as hypoglycaemia is more likely. Although patients with infarction may vomit at presentation or secondary to opiate administration, this usually settles with antiemetics and may not interfere with oral therapy.

A recent study did not identify a blood glucose level above which complications developed in the diabetic patient with infarction (Gwilt et al, 1984), and one has to rely on clinical judgement of what is reasonable. Probably a blood glucose of 12 mmol/l or above on more than one occasion should indicate oral therapy for the patient on diet alone or insulin for the patient on maximal oral therapy. Clearly a short-acting sulphonylurea such as tolbutamide or a medium-acting one such as glibenclamide is particularly useful in this situation.

If insulin is required a convenient regime is to use a highly purified porcine or human short-acting insulin subcutaneously. A single dose may be needed to reduce a markedly elevated blood glucose and then glycaemic control may be maintained with twice-daily injections. In some cases it may be necessary to resort to three or four injections of short-acting insulin. The dietitian will need to be informed so that regular amounts of carbohydrate can be provided in a suitable form.

When the patient is over the acute episode and begins recovery the insulin requirement usually decreases. A decision can then be taken whether to revert to oral agents or continue with insulin. If the latter course is chosen the patient can either be transferred to a once-daily insulin regime with a long-acting insulin or alternatively a twice-daily regime perhaps with a fixed combination of short- and intermediate-acting insulin. If the patient is left on insulin following discharge from hospital the question of continuing insulin therapy can be reviewed in the diabetic clinic. Clearly it is important to review all these patients after discharge from hospital and decide their long-term management.

A minority of patients will run a very stormy course after admission with myocardial infarction complicated perhaps by arrhythmias, severe heart failure and reinfarction. They will be maximally stressed and probably able to take little orally due to vomiting and/or impaired gastrointestinal absorption. Under these circumstances an intravenous infusion of insulin provides a very convenient and reliable method for managing the diabetes. The principal limitation to intravenous therapy with insulin is the availability of skilled and diligent nursing staff to ensure that the apparatus is correctly set up, the infusion rate is as instructed and the insulin is infused into the patient. However, on a coronary care unit with adequate, trained and qualified staff this is not usually a problem. Highly purified procine or human short-acting insulin is added to a small volume of normal saline and infused using a pump set at a rate dependent on blood glucose monitoring. The blood glucose should be monitored hourly after commencing an intravenous insulin infusion to ensure that the patient is not becoming hypoglycaemic. This may not be obvious clinically in a sedated poorly perfused patient with a complicated infarction. Once a satisfactory level is achieved then blood glucose monitoring can be extended initially to two-hourly. At least one major centre is using a continuous intravenous insulin infusion for all diabetics with infarcts (Lamb, 1984).

For patients with complicated infarctions requiring intensive insulin therapy the recovery phase will be heralded by a diminishing insulin requirement. At this stage it is convenient to change to an insulin regimen intermediate between the intravenous infusion and the relaxed regimen of one or two injections per day in the well patient. Six-hourly subcutaneous injections of highly purified short-acting insulin usually meet the requirements and are continued for one or two days before the final transition is made to the patient's customary insulin regimen.

Sliding scales should be mentioned at this point. They tend to be frowned upon by those caring for diabetic patients. They are frequently written in a way that omits insulin when the blood glucose is within the normal range, and they usually fail to take account of the insulin resistance induced by increased ketone body production. Occasionally diabetic patients can become severely ketotic without being very hyperglycaemic. The most important principle of insulin therapy in the insulin-dependent patient is that insulin must be given regularly to inhibit lipolysis and prevent ketosis. The foregoing is summarised in Figure 6.1.

Who should look after the diabetic patients on the coronary care unit or the intensive therapy unit? I believe all doctors and nurses using these units are more than capable of managing most of the diabetic problems. The role of the physician with an interest in diabetes is to ensure that they have the necessary treatment policies and training and that he is readily available for advice on the more difficult cases.

To Reduce the Risk of Coronary Artery Disease

One of the most important aims of modern diabetic care must be to delay the onset of chronic complications by optimal management. Let us consider why careful management may be beneficial.

We have evidence from studies on non-diabetics that treating hypertension reduces the incidence of stroke, congestive cardiac failure and possibly myocardial infarction (Veterans Administration Co-operative Study Group on

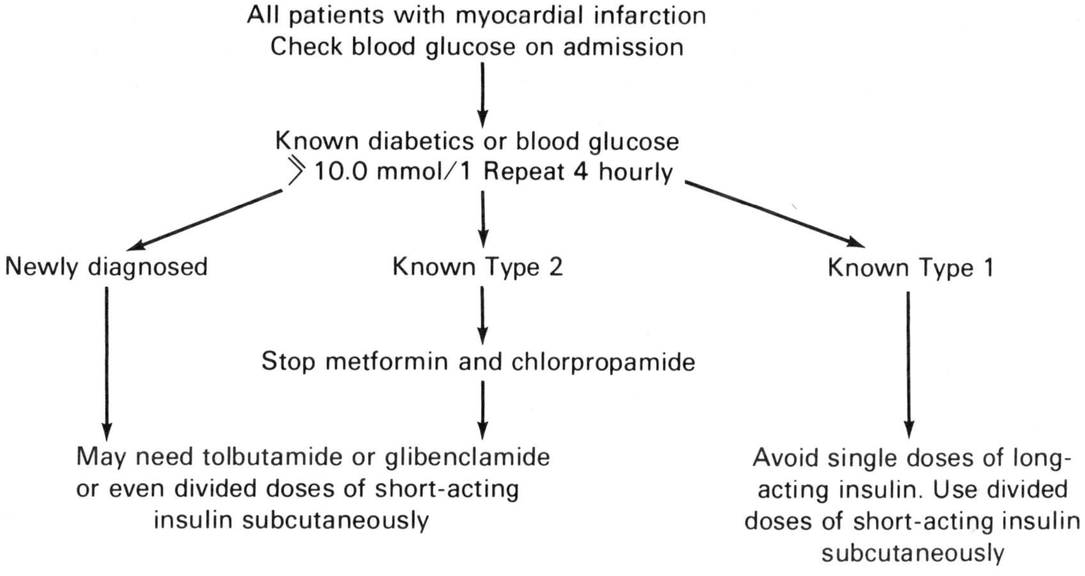

Figure 6.1 The management of the blood glucose during myocardial infarction.

Antihypertensive Agents, 1967, 1970; Hypertension Detection and Follow-Up Program, 1979). Studies on serum cholesterol levels in non-diabetics have shown that a degree of primary prevention of coronary artery disease is achieved by lowering serum cholesterol levels in high-risk populations of males with significant hypercholesterolaemia using diet and drug treatment (The Lipid Research Clinics Coronary Primary Prevention Trial, 1984) or diet alone (Hjermann et al, 1981). Hypertension and hypercholesterolaemia are common accompaniments of diabetes and it is not illogical to anticipate similar benefits if these atherogenic factors are dealt with effectively in the diabetic patient.

Hyperglycaemia *per se* is an important factor predisposing to atheroma, possibly via an effect on platelet aggregation or on structural proteins comprising the tissues of the arterial wall or by mechanisms unknown. There have been no studies yet in diabetics showing that a group with really good glycaemic control has a lower incidence of coronary artery disease than a well-matched control group. Such studies will be difficult to mount because they will need large numbers of patients followed over many years to demonstrate any benefit. It is surely unjustifiable not to provide optimal control of blood glucose in the rest of the diabetic population while the results of these studies are awaited, provided that the means of achieving optimal glycaemic control are acceptable to patients, free from undesirable effects and not unduly expensive.

Three major steps forward in diabetic care in this century have been the discovery of insulin, the development of treatment programmes for diabetic ketoacidosis and the management of pregnancy in the diabetic patient. This latter breakthrough brought together diabetologist and obstetrician to produce comprehensive care, with improved glycaemic control contributing to dramatic decreases in perinatal mortality and morbidity (Karlsson & Kjellmer, 1972). I suspect that we are about to witness a similar phenomenon with regard to the chronic complications of diabetes, including coronary artery disease, due to comprehensive patient care with special emphasis on control of blood glucose, blood pressure, lipids and a decline in the prevalence of cigarette smoking.

Type 1 Diabetes

This type of diabetes is diagnosed usually in the first half of life, exposing those affected to abnormal levels of blood glucose and other metabolites for decades. Many of these individuals will lose their remaining endogenous insulin secretion as β-cell destruction progresses, becoming wholly dependent on exogenous insulin with the associated problems of more difficult glycaemic control.

A prime requirement for the prevention of chronic complications such as coronary heart disease appears to be good glycaemic control, because many associated abnormalities such as hyperlipidaemia (Sosenko et al, 1980) and perhaps increased platelet aggregation (Petersen et al, 1977) may be improved as the blood glucose level is normalised. Undoubtedly the ideal solutions would be (1) preservation of significant β-cell function by selectively suppressing immunological destruction permitting at least some degree of physiological glucose homeostasis or (2) a miniature insulin pump that would infuse insulin subcutaneously, regulated by a sensor indicating the tissue fluid glucose level together with a suitably programmed microprocessor system. Both these approaches are being actively investigated and one day we may see a revolution in management of Type 1 diabetes. For the moment we have to rely on intermittent subcutaneous injections which impose quite definite restrictions. If the same dose and type of insulin are given at the same time each day and either the food intake or the amount of physical activity fluctuates to a significant degree, the consequences are going to be unacceptable hyperglycaemia or hypoglycaemia. In the not-too-distant past the attitude of physicians was very much to avoid even the suggestion of hypoglycaemic reactions at any time, and always to keep a little glucose in the urine, especially at bedtime.

The diabetic clinic of those days did not even have blood glucose results available when patients were seen: now most clinics enjoy this advance. Two more recent developments have been home blood glucose monitoring and the glycosylated haemoglobin (HbA_1) or fructosamine — indicators of the integrated blood glucose level over the preceding few weeks. Home monitoring is now possible using test strips either in conjunction with a meter or simply using visual assessment. The real advantage with this development is that the patient can now start to appreciate how the blood glucose varies with diet, exercise and illness. Measuring the blood glucose at home will not in itself result in improved glycaemic control. The patient must understand the achievable range of blood glucose and have the knowledge and confidence to attain that range consistently by balancing the dose of insulin with diet, exercise and intercurrent illness. We are expecting much more of patients than in the past. Undoubtedly some will be unable to cope with this emphasis on self-management because they lack either the intelligence or perhaps, more importantly, the motivation to do so. For those who are capable of learning how to modify diet and insulin dose to suit prevailing circumstances and want to do so, the ability to determine their own blood glucose has been a major step forward, permitting more satisfactory glycaemic control and a more adventurous approach to many activities (Skyler et al, 1978; Sonksen et al, 1978; Walford et al, 1978).

The other important development has been the glycosylated haemoglobin level. This gives an indication of the ambient blood glucose level over the previous two or three months and is the best single indicator we have at present of glycaemic control. We can now classify patients as having good or bad glycaemic control. More importantly, we can supply patients with their results so that they can see how effective their personal management has been. If the result is unsatisfactory it can be used as a motivating factor to persuade them to try and make an improvement. Serum fructosamine concentration looks a possible alternative to HbA_1 (Baker et al, 1985): it is reliable and reflects the integrated blood glucose level over three to six weeks versus eight to 12. Advantages of fructosamine are that it does not depend on the haemoglobin level and it will probably be considerably cheaper.

The principal aim of the modern diabetic clinic must be to prevent complications, and therefore it needs to be organised so that Type 1 patients can be motivated and educated successfully to manage their diabetes. A programme of teaching is required, taking place outside the diabetic clinic at times convenient to the patients, avoiding loss of time from school and work. The programme needs to be practical so that patients can apply what they have learned to their own situations. It needs to cover the essentials of self-management: diet, insulin, type and duration of action, injection timing and technique, measuring blood glucose and the normal range, hypoglycaemia, exercise and illness. It should include assessment and provide feedback on progress with glycosylated haemoglobin levels.

Diet

It was in the late 1970s that the potential hazards of traditional carbohydrate restriction were fully realised. Carbohydrate restriction had been used in the preinsulin era to try to control hyperglycaemia. When insulin was introduced its use in less severe form was continued with the intention of keeping the dose of insulin down and controlling the blood glucose. The hazard of this diet was that patients had to have an alternative source of energy so they turned to fat. Foods such as fatty meats, cheese, cream and butter were often eaten in liberal amounts. These foods contain saturated fat and cholesterol and their effect is to tend to increase the serum cholesterol (McGill et al, 1968; Keys, 1970). Diabetics tend to have higher serum cholesterol levels than non-diabetes (Santen et al, 1972), and the old diabetic diet only recently abandoned may have been a contributing factor. Enthusiasm for a change in dietary recommendations for diabetic patients was fuelled by growing awareness of links between the serum cholesterol level and coronary heart disease, and dietary fat intake and serum cholesterol in the non-diabetic population. Suddenly the inadvisability of having an atheroma-prone group on a high-fat diet was fully recognised. The diet currently recommended for diabetics in the UK is relatively low in fat and high in unrefined carbohydrate and fibre (British Diabetic Association, 1982). The diet should have a beneficial effect on blood lipids without contributing to hyperglycaemia.

If attitudes to the content of the diabetic diet have changed radically, the importance of the regularity of meals and snacks is as important as ever for the patient on intermittent injections of insulin. Now that the aim is to keep the young diabetic's blood glucose in single figures as much as possible, the risk of hypoglycaemia is increased and there is much less latitude for missing breakfast after a late night or delaying a meal. This is probably one of the most difficult factors for the young diabetic to accept and undoubtedly a great advantage of continuous subcutaneous insulin infusion is that it permits the patient greater flexibility in relation to the timing of meals with manual boluses of insulin 30 minutes beforehand.

Perhaps the greatest single problem with diet as an instrument of therapy is persuading patients to comply with it. There are three ingredients required for successful compliance: first, the patient must be motivated to comply; second, he must be informed about diet in a way that is individually appropriate; thirdly, realistic and attainable objectives must be set. The patient is then rewarded by achieving these objectives and motivation is enhanced. The motivational ingredient is the most difficult. Successful motivation depends on emphasising positive tangible benefits. Promises such as 'you will avoid complications' or 'live longer' may be grasped with enthusiasm by the over-forties but are unlikely to appeal to youngsters. Informing appropriately has been neglected in the past. Diet used to be taught by personal interview and printed diet sheet. It is odd that doctors accepted this approach because as medical students we were never taught in this way, rather by demonstration and participation. To make matters worse many dietary instructional leaflets required a reading age not attained by the target population.

The old way to teach about an aspect of diet, say party-eating at Christmas, would be to discuss it and hand out a leaflet. The modern way is to meet a group of patients over a party-type meal and discuss how to cope with the problems that may arise. Experienced diabetic patients make good practical teachers. Hopefully this approach may avoid the extremes of complete abandonment of dietary principles on the one hand and obsessional self-denial on the other.

Insulin

A very important advance has been highly purified insulin, and more recently we have had human insulin from recombinant DNA which will probably become the major source of the world's insulin in the future. We have insulins which cover a wide range of duration of action, but we still have injections which must be the least palatable aspect of life for the patient requiring insulin.

A patient commencing insulin needs to be taught and to learn about the equipment, its care and storage, drawing up insulin, injection technique, sites to use and timing of injections. This is the easy part, proving difficult only for those with unsteady hands, poor vision or failure to comprehend. More difficult is conveying that injections must be self-administered and must not be missed. Self-administration is important because it implies the acceptance by the patient that he has diabetes and realises the importance of self-reliance. Most people caring for diabetic patients realise the importance of the patient actively participating in the very first injection of insulin. It is symbolic of the attitude that injecting insulin need not be frightening or difficult and can be coped with by the patient from the very beginning, with just a little guidance. Failure to achieve this goal at the outset may result in a patient who depends on others for insulin injections, misses injections or does them with a very poor technique. The result is an unhappy patient and poor glycaemic control.

The answer to the question 'which insulin regime?' must be 'the one which produces the most satisfactory glycaemic control over 24 hours'. There is no virtue in several injections of insulin if the patient is well controlled on a single injection each day, but this state of affairs is unlikely to be the case in a patient who has had diabetes for a number of years and has little residual β-cell function. It is probably better psychological strategy to start the newly insulin-requiring patient on two injections of insulin per day so that there is early acceptance of this regimen. Bringing a group of patients together is a useful way of getting patients currently content with one injection a day to enquire why they are not having two injections a day as are the other patients they have met.

We are spoilt for choice with insulins. There are highly purified porcine and bovine varieties, human insulin synthesised from porcine insulin (semi-synthetic) and human insulin from recombinant DNA (biosynthetic). The one subject on which there seems to be unanimity, is that purity of insulin has been an important advance (Andreani et al, 1977). Species of insulin is less important although there may be advantages in using porcine rather than bovine insulin (Clark et al, 1982). Interestingly, there is no convincing evidence that human insulin is preferable to porcine (Home & Alberti, 1982). This explains the reluctance of many clinicians in the UK to change patients from porcine to semi-synthetic or biosynthetic human insulin. Any trend towards human insulin might increase if the price were to decrease below that of porcine insulin.

There is considerable individual variation with regard to insulin requirement. Most will need two injections of intermediate-acting insulin a day with some short-acting to cover breakfast, a mid-morning snack and lunch. Theoretically short-acting insulin in the evening would cover the evening meal and bedtime snack, but some patients readily become hypoglycaemic with short-acting insulin at this time. The dawn phenomenon — rising blood glucose due to an increased insulin requirement in the early morning — is seen in most diabetics and presents practical problems in a few (Bolli & Gerich, 1984, Editorial, 1984). This may be the cause of marked prebreakfast hyperglycaemia sometimes with ketonuria. A stratagem that may solve this problem is to give short-acting insulin alone before the evening meal and intermediate-acting insulin at bedtime (Tattersall & Gale, 1981; Francis et al, 1983). The dawn phenomenon may also be successfully controlled in patients receiving infusions of insulin, although the nocturnal infusion rate may need modification (Geffner et al, 1983; Levy-Marchal et al, 1983; Bending et al, 1984).

Another method of producing 24-hour glycaemic control is to use a very long-acting insulin (36 hours) injected before breakfast to provide the baseline insulin and supplement it with injections of short-acting insulin before breakfast and the evening meal (Phillips et al, 1979). It may have a wider application with the advent of 'pen' syringes now available utilising cartridges for short-acting insulin. Depression of the plunger delivers two units of insulin obviating the need for drawing up and simplifying the procedure for when patients are out and about. A third injection of short-acting insulin can be added at midday if required. Suggestions that this can lead to relaxation of the guiding principles of regular rations and insulin are disquieting.

A very useful development in insulin therapy in recent years has been the fixed-dose mixture of insulin, either 30 per cent short-acting and 70 per cent intermediate-acting (Mixtard) or equal parts of the two insulins (Initard). Another insulin manufacturer has now produced a fixed mixture of insulins very similar to Mixtard, called Actraphane. It is only available as a semisynthetic human insulin, whereas at present there are porcine and semisynthetic preparations of Mixtard. Evidence is accumulating that probably less benefit is achieved by juggling with proportions of short- and intermediate-acting insulin than was previously thought (Roland, 1984). The fixed dose mixtures are certainly useful for patients who are unable or unwilling to draw up two different insulins.

Only recently has the importance of the timing of insulin injections in relation to meals become fully realised. This applies to patients taking short-acting insulin to cover meals and snacks. The best results are obtained if insulin is administered at least 30 minutes before the meal (Lean et al, 1985). This leads to lower postprandial glucose levels and less frequent episodes of hypoglycaemia.

A most useful exercise in the diabetic clinic is inspection of injection sites. Many patients habitually use one or two sites and develop hard subcutaneous plaques or disfiguring insulin hypertrophy. It is fruitless asking patients if their injection sites are satisfactory, as they invariably say that they are; they come to regard the abnormal as normal. Absorption from such sites is very likely to be erratic, leading to poorly controlled diabetes and possibly unexplained hypoglycaemia.

How much insulin does a patient need? Enough to keep him ketone-free with single-figure blood glucose levels most of the time, at as near ideal body weight as possible and avoiding hypoglycaemia. The most common pitfall in managing insulin-requiring diabetes is to respond to elevated blood glucose levels by increasing the dose of insulin. Certain key aspects need to be reviewed before increasing the dose of insulin, including diet, injection technique and condition of injection sites. A most undesirable feature is the production of an obese diabetic by inappropriately increasing the insulin dose and failing to detect latent hypoglycaemia. Insulin dose needs to be titrated against the results of home monitoring of blood glucose levels, a careful search for evidence of hypoglycaemia and a continuous record of bodyweight.

Continuous subcutaneous infusion of insulin

This can be a very effective method of achieving good glycaemic control for diabetic patients requiring insulin (Mecklenburg et al, 1982, 1985). Patients need to be carefully selected so that they are sensible and responsible. It is particularly appropriate for young patients with diabetes of only a few years' duration and without complications. Significant retinopathy is a contraindication as it may deteriorate with greatly improved glycaemic control (Lauritzen et al, 1983). Patients with brittle diabetes or recurrent staphylococcal infections are also unsuitable for infusion pumps. Patients need intensive education in the use of the pump and changing the needle and infusion set. The pump delivers a continuous but adjustable basal rate and boluses can be given before meals. It is essential that patients ensure there are no leaks of insulin where the infusion set is connected to the syringe. They need to be able to measure accurately their blood glucose and test the urine for ketones when unwell. It is a wise precaution for them to carry conventional insulins and have a regimen organised should they be troubled by pump failure. It is also essential that they have a telephone number where diabetic expertise is continuously available. It is not advisable to let patients travel outside the country with a pump. How long should a patient use a pump? This is not an easy question to answer. A very useful role for the pump is to determine more accurately the patient's insulin requirement, and improve the patient's understanding of the effect of diet, insulin, exercise and minor illness on the blood glucose. A useful scheme is to try the patient on a conventional insulin regime after three to six months on a pump.

Home monitoring

The time-honoured method has been by urine testing, but with the renal threshold in the not so elderly being of the order of 10 mmol/l glycosuria is only going to occur when the blood glucose is in double figures. This method is perhaps more acceptable for those who cannot or will not cope with blood testing or who have very stable diabetes because of some residual β-cell function. Blood testing enables patients to see how their diet, exercise, illnesses and insulin affect the blood glucose. They can confirm or refute the idea that they may be hypoglycaemic. Initially a meter was thought to be desirable for accurate monitoring, but now there are available test strips which do not require a meter and are sufficiently accurate for the purpose if correctly used (Ferguson & Prosser, 1980).

Patients do not need to home monitor every day when their diabetes is stable but rather two or three days a week testing three or four times during the day. If it is to be of maximum benefit they must be able to perform monitoring correctly, interpret the results and use the information to modify diet or insulin dose as appropriate. Not all patients on insulin will benefit from regular home monitoring. Particularly suitable candidates are those with unstable diabetes and evidence of poor control with elevated glycosylated haemoglobin levels.

Type 2 Diabetes

This is more prevalent than Type 1 and usually presents in the over-forties. It is often associated with obesity and may be latent for some years before diagnosis. Patients often have concomitant hypertension and at the time of diagnosis may already have angina and claudication. There is a strong familial component to this type of diabetes and perhaps ideally the primary medical care service should provide an annual postprandial blood glucose test for those over 40 years with a first-degree relative who has developed diabetes before the age of 65 years. This might reduce the length of exposure to the

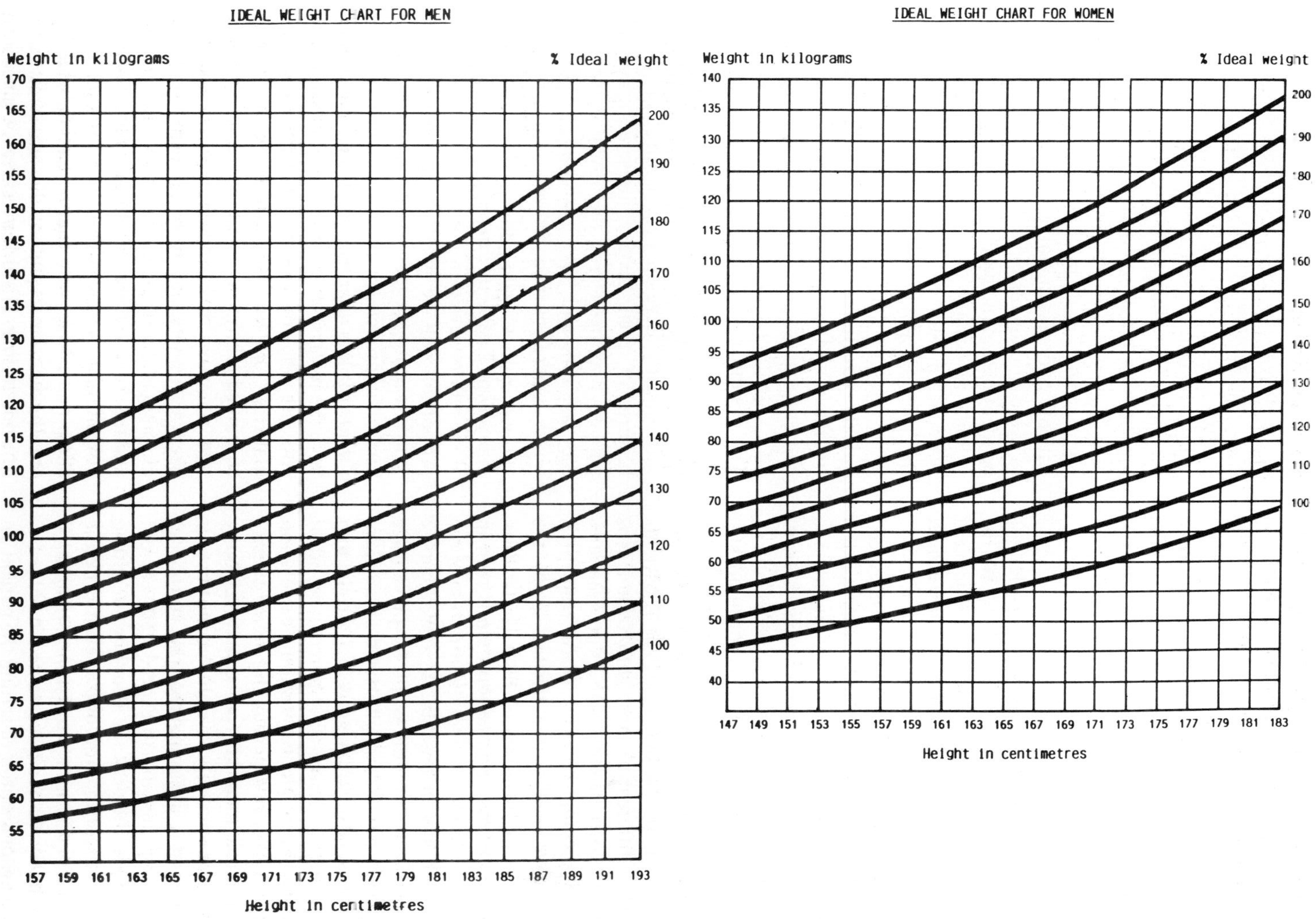

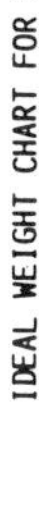

Figure 6.2 Data obtained from Metropolitan Life Insurance Company Statistical Bulletin 40, Nov–Dec 1959. Medium frame size was used and the mean weights of the ranges taken as ideal weight. Patients weighed and measured without shoes or outdoor clothing.

atherogenic factors of hyperglycaemia and disordered lipid metabolism. The single most useful measure for preventing Type 2 diabetes in the industrialised nations would be a reduction in energy intake with a consequent reduction in the prevalence of obesity, hyperlipidaemia, glucose intolerance and possibly hypertension.

Diet

The importance of diet in this group of patients is that for some diet alone will suffice, while for the rest there must be a good dietary compliance if control is to be optimal at a steady weight whether using oral agents or insulin.

Regularity of meals remains important, especially for the obese. Many of these patients claim that they cannot be fat because they eat only one meal a day. This meal may of course be of gargantuan proportions and much snacking of high-energy foods may precede its consumption. Three regular meals a day avoiding snacks often leads to weight reduction.

The content of the diet for Type 2 patients need not be different to those with Type 1. It is helpful to classify patients with Type 2 diabetes into obese and non-obese. A useful concept is that of ideal bodyweight derived from the Metropolitan Life Insurance tables. The data are based on a different population than is seen in British clinics but it provides quantitation of the degree of obesity in practice. In our clinic we have constructed a centile graph for percentage ideal or desirable bodyweight based on medium frame size, so that knowing actual weight and height we can derive the percentage ideal bodyweight at a glance without calculation (Figure 6.2). We are generous and define obesity as being more than 120 per cent ideal body weight. Selecting a target weight for the obese is important and it is essential that this is realistic. It is counter-productive to expect a 50-year-old patient who is 160 per cent ideal bodyweight to join the ranks of the non-obese; even if heroic efforts achieve this miraculous transformation, it is very unlikely it could be sustained for 20 years. It is once again a matter of setting the patient an achievable and sustainable objective. In this case if our 50-year-old reduced his weight by a stone or so and maintained it indefinitely it may well be enough to control the diabetes.

For the non-obese patients, simply reducing the intake of refined carbohydrate may control the diabetes for a time at least. These patients may be at or below their ideal bodyweight so it is important they do not lose more weight. Some patients may try to starve themselves in order to avoid oral agents or insulin, and this needs to be identified immediately.

Some physicians devalue dietary therapy for Type 2 diabetes by either commencing oral therapy concomitantly with diet or by giving diet alone no more than a month's trial. The patient quickly concludes that tablets are the real treatment and the diet of secondary importance. Not surprisingly they may consequently pay it little attention and even discard it altogether. The results of this approach are that some individuals may be committed to lifelong drug therapy which they do not need. Others may subsequently develop poor control on tablets because of their dietary indiscretions. Some patients may need drug therapy at diagnosis if they are thin and have lost much weight with severe hyperglycaemia, are very symptomatic or perhaps with evidence of infection. However, many Type 2 patients can be commenced on diet alone and reviewed in a month. A considerable proportion will be greatly improved and it is worth waiting another couple of months to see further improvement before commencing drug therapy. If this approach is effective the patients have the reward of feeling better for their efforts and see the relationship between diet and diabetes. This provides valuable motivation to continued effort.

A point worth making here is that patients need to understand from an early stage the meaning of diabetes, that they have diabetes now and that they will always have it. The following is not unusual. A new patient attends the diabetic clinic and is informed that he has diabetes. He sees the dietitian, is put on a diet and is instructed in urine testing. His urine tests show glycosuria which over the months abates. He feels that he is cured now and stops testing. He gradually forgets about the diet. This pitfall can be avoided by ensuring that the subject is covered in an educational programme and by providing long-term follow-up with a system that seeks out those who do not attend the clinic.

Oral agents

There is still considerable debate about the role of tablets in the treatment of Type 2 diabetes. When they were introduced they offered an alternative to insulin for the patient not responding to diet alone. A study was later published which seemed to indicate that patients on tablets had a higher mortality from coronary heart disease than other groups not receiving oral therapy (University Group Diabetes Program 1970). A criticism of these data was that the groups were not comparable and that this difference could have accounted for the results rather than the effects of therapy. Later work from a retrospective study suggested that sulphonylurea therapy may reduce levels of high-density lipoprotein cholesterol (Kennedy et al, 1978). A subsequent prospective study demonstrated that neither metformin nor glibenclamide had an adverse effect on serum total cholesterol, triglyceride, HDL-cholesterol or the apoproteins A-I and B (Taylor et al, 1982).

The introduction of biguanides was met with some scepticism of their efficacy and fears about the possibility of precipitating lactic acidosis. Later it was realised that this problem was particularly associated with phenformin and, provided metformin is avoided in the presence of renal or hepatic impairment, tissue hypoxia or significant ketone body production, it is safe (Bergman et al, 1978; Luft et al, 1978; Nattrass & Alberti, 1978). Phenformin has subsequently been withdrawn from the register of prescribable drugs in the UK.

More has been learned about the mechanisms of action of the two oral hypoglycaemic families of drugs — the sulphonylureas and the biguan-

ides. The sulphonylureas increase plasma insulin levels in patients in whom they are effective and they may also enhance tissue sensitivity to insulin via a postreceptor effect (Lockwood et al, 1984). Metformin lowers blood glucose not by an effect on insulin secretion but by inhibiting hepatic gluconeogenesis, possibly increasing peripheral low-affinity insulin receptors, and it may exert a postreceptor effect (Lord et al, 1983; Lockwood et al ,1984).

One distinct advantage of metformin over the sulphonylureas in obese Type 2 patients is that it does tend to suppress appetite and certainly therapy is usually associated with weight loss (Taylor et al, 1982). Disadvantages with metformin are that a minority of patients may develop a metallic taste in the mouth, indigestion or loose bowel actions. These side-effects may be avoided by using only 500-mg tablets with a maximum of three per day taken after meals. Some patients do not complain of the side-effects or relate them to therapy, so it is worth questioning patients carefully to see that all is well. Successful therapy is measured by a loss of glycosuria, blood glucose levels less than 10.0 mmol/l postprandially and a glycosylated haemoglobin of 10.0 per cent or less. If this is not achieved with diet and metformin then the alternatives are adding in a guar gum preparation or a sulphonylurea. Guar gum is a complex polysaccharide which cannot be digested or absorbed and it appears to have two effects. First, it takes up water and swells after ingestion so, taken before meals, it exerts a satiating effect and may decrease energy intake. Secondly, it seems to reduce glucose absorption in the small intestine (Blackburn et al, 1984). There are a number of reasonably palatable preparations of guar now available.

If guar gum proves ineffective or unpalatable then a sulphonylurea can be added, preferably avoiding the excessively long-acting chloropropamide. If an obese diabetic patient has poor glycaemic control with steady or increasing bodyweight, the explanation is one of non-compliance with diet. This situation is very difficult to handle and it is worth trying to avoid early escalation of treatment with sulphony-lureas and then progressing to insulin. It is important to ascertain why dietary compliance is poor. It may be lack of understanding of the appropriate diet or an inability to put it into practice. One can try very hard on an outpatient basis to inform the patient and other members of the family, particularly the spouse. We often admit patients with this problem to the diabetic unit for a few days to demonstrate how effective the right diet can be. This also gives a good opportunity to educate about diet and test that knowledge in practical terms as well as enhancing motivation to comply.

If obese Type 2 patients who are not complying with diet are given sulphonylureas which stimulate insulin secretion or insulin itself, the consequences are all too frequently an even more obese patient with glycaemic control still very poor — a very undesirable situation. It is essential that this group of patients grasp the essential dietary principles at the outset.

For the non-obese Type 2 patient reducing the intake of refined carbohydrate may be effective, but many may need to progress to a sulphony-lurea with intermediate duration of action such as glibenclamide. Frequently patients respond to a small dose and indeed some patients may be very sensitive to this drug and care needs to be taken that hypoglycaemia does not occur. For this reason it is prudent to commence with the smallest dose of glibenclamide, namely 2.5 mg. Patients need to be cautioned about not missing meals and using alcohol with discretion when receiving sulphonylureas because of the risk of precipitating hypoglycaemia.

If a patient has lost much weight and particularly if underweight, then a good case can be made for commencing insulin. The other indication for insulin is of course when glycaemic control is poor on a maximal dose of a sulphony-lurea. Sometimes metformin is added to sul-phonylurea therapy, usually because the patient is having difficulty coming to terms with the prospect of insulin. It is very easy for the physician to fail to appreciate how poorly controlled some Type 2 patients really are.

Patients may only record negative urine testing results in the preprandial state and starve themselves before the diabetic clinic. This is an area which has been generally illuminated by the glycosylated haemoglobin level which gives a much surer guide of the true state of glycaemic control.

For the non-obese patient over 65 years who needs a sulphonylurea, a short-acting drug like tolbutamide has much to commend it as the elderly are more prone to hypoglycaemia. If this drug fails to control the diabetes than a more potent preparation such as glibenclamide may be required. A case can be made for giving tolbutamide to those 65 years and over who are obese Type 2 patients and need an oral agent. The reasoning here is that renal function tends to decline with age and renal elimination is important in preventing accumulation of metfor-min, at least theoretically increasing the risk of lactic acidosis (Luft et al, 1978).

Insulin therapy

When a Type 2 patient requires insulin, perhaps the first question to ask is 'One or two injections a day?' The answer depends partly on the age of the patient. It is always difficult to choose an arbitrary age but perhaps under 60 years two injections and over 60 one injection. The implication is that two injections are better than one, which is not always true, and that less strict glycaemic control is acceptable with a shorter expected lifespan, which seems reasonable. Although two injections a day may be desirable the next question is whether it is possible. This depends on the patient's eyesight, manual dexterity and willingness. For those commencing two daily injections, the fixed insulin combina-tions can be very useful as older patients often find mixing insulins a difficult exercise. How-ever, for patients in their forties it is usually a simple matter to establish them on similar insulin regimens to the Type 1 patients.

For the over sixties a once-daily insulin will often produce satisfactory control. However, if control is very poor in spite of a satisfactory diet with a single daily dose of c.50 units of insulin, it is better to consider two injections rather than increasing the dose. Before resorting to this it is worth ensuring that the injection technique is satisfactory and the injection sites are healthy.

It is too easy to assume that older patients cannot inject their own insulin and thus need to involve relatives or the district nurse. The best approach is for the patient to be totally independent if at all possible. The second best is under the watchful eye or with the help of a relative. Using a person outside the family circle, such as the district nurse, is positively the last resort. It is undesirable because the patient is totally dependent on someone coming into the home from outside and of course it is extremely expensive in terms of nursing time.

The following questions need answering when deciding if the patient can become independent with their injections. (1) Is the eyesight adequate to see the marks on the syringe? Sometimes this can be helped by a magnifier fitted to the syringe, or a separate magnifying glass. (2) Can the patient remember to have the injection and the correct dose? Someone living with the patient may be able to remind them of these points. (3) Does the patient have the manual dexterity to draw up the insulin and inject it? Keeping the regimen simple is important, so that mixing of insulin is not required. If two injections are required, attempting to use the same dose morning and evening may be helpful. Fixed-dose syringes can be very useful, and perhaps a relative can draw up the insulin and the patient administer it.

Monitoring control

Many patients with Type 2 diabetes retain some degree of endogenous insulin production, and this may explain their tendency to have more stable blood glucose levels in contrast to patients with Type 1 diabetes. Consequently, Type 2 patients do not need to assess control quite as frequently as the Type 1 patients once good glycaemic control has been achieved. For patients on diet alone a check on the blood glucose and glycosylated haemoglobin by the general practitioner or diabetic clinic will suffice, with the patient testing the urine for glucose twice weekly avoiding using early-morning specimens. This needs emphasising to patients, as some on diet alone quickly learn that they have glycosuria after meals so solve the problem by testing the urine after the overnight fast or before meals. This is an interesting example of the patient learning what is expected (no glycosuria) but adopting the wrong solution. The correct approach is dietary modification or, if that is satisfactory, oral agents so that there is no postprandial glycosuria. Indications for home monitoring of blood glucose in these patients are a raised glycosylated haemoglobin or a low renal threshold.

The glycosylated haemoglobin has been a very useful advance for the Type 2 patients with latently poor control. These patients may be on diet alone or diet and oral agents with records of urine results which they have continually mislaid. The blood glucose level checked by the practice nurse or diabetic clinic is perhaps just in single figures but with close questioning the patient has had very little to eat for several hours. The glycosylated haemoglobin result is markedly elevated, revealing the extent of poor control. Useful clinical pointers are the unavailability for various reasons of the patient's urine tests — lost book, came out in a hurry, left it on the bus — occurring with each clinic visit, and an enquiry as to when the patient last had something to eat. Some patients regard diabetic clinic days as holy days and fast for them!

Hypertension

This is more common in diabetic patients and is an important causative factor of coronary artery disease in its own right. It is stating the obvious, but regular measurement of blood pressure using the correct technique is an essential feature of good diabetic care. Regularly means annually for normotensive patients and more frequently for the known hypertensives. If blood pressure is elevated the first question must be 'Am I using the correct size cuff?' If the circumference of the upper arm is 33 cm or more a large cuff should be used (Maxwell et al, 1982). The diagnosis of hypertension requires more than one reading. Additional reasons for checking the blood pressure are marked retinopathy or any evidence of proteinuria. Having measured the blood pressure it is essential to record it prominently and if hypertension is diagnosed to ensure it is adequately treated. It is extremely worrying that in non-diabetics half the cases of hypertension are undiagnosed, half those diagnosed are untreated and of the half that are treated half are inadequately controlled (WHO Expert Committee on Hypertension, 1978). There is no reason to believe that diabetic patients fare better and they may do less well.

With regard to treatment, this subject has already been covered in some detail. An important principle of treatment is that it should control the hypertension to an acceptable degree, be free from side-effects and not cause either an unacceptable deterioration of glycaemic control or have an adverse effect on blood lipids. An unacceptable deterioration of glycaemic control occurs when control cannot readily be restored by a minor alteration of the treatment regimen. To control blood pressure at the expense of the blood glucose level or with elevated lipid levels does not represent successful treatment.

Lipids

If hypertension has been neglected in the diabetic care of the past, lipids might not have existed for the attention they have received.

Occasionally hyperlipidaemia may be overt with eruptive xanthomata, lipaemia retinalis or lipaemic serum which blocks the autoanalyser and causes pseudohyponatraemia. Usually it is covert and can only be diagnosed by specifically measuring blood lipids.

A problem with diagnosing lipid disorders is that everyone has been obsessed with examining fasting specimens, a requirement which presents two obstacles for diabetics. Firstly, it requires an extra visit to the hospital and, secondly, fasting is difficult for the patient on insulin. There is not a great difference between the serum cholesterol level in the fasting or in the fed state and it is certainly worth using a random cholesterol as a screening test. If this is satisfactory then no further action is required, as the fasting cholesterol will be lower than the random determination. Serum triglyceride levels are more affected by the ingestion of food, but one quickly learns to gauge what amounts to satisfactory random cholesterol and triglyceride results and when a fasting specimen is required. The right time to measure lipids for the newly diagnosed diabetic is when good control has been achieved and thereafter probably yearly up to the age of sixty.

The treatment of hyperlipidaemia in the diabetic patient falls into three natural stages: (1) control of the diabetes by appropriate diet and oral agents or insulin if necessary; (2) reassessment of the diet if hyperlipidaemia persists; (3) drug therapy only when the diabetes and the diet are right.

Smoking

There are few studies on the prevalence of smoking in diabetics but one from the West of Scotland suggests there is little difference compared to their non-diabetic fellows (Kesson & Slater, 1979). This reflects badly on those involved with diabetic care because it suggests that not enough attention has been devoted to discouraging this atherogenic activity in an atheroma-prone group. A major problem is that those caring for patients are only too well aware of the restrictions they are tending to impose. Patients are advised to eat regular meals, avoid certain foods, take tablets or inject themselves with insulin, monitor their blood glucose levels, to be careful with alcohol and see their doctors regularly. Many physicians regard giving antismoking advice as just too much and this falls by the wayside. Although understandable, this attitude cannot be condoned. Perhaps the best approach is to devise methods by which patients conclude for themselves that smoking is harmful and undesirable. Self-help groups can be very useful and ideally every physician caring for diabetics should have access to a person skilled in helping people to rid themselves of the smoking habit.

Who Should be Responsible for Diabetic Care?

For many years there has been much debate in the UK about who should care for diabetic patients — general practitioners or hospital-based doctors. This question has been answered to some extent by a recent paper which showed a significantly higher mortality and morbidity among diabetics discharged solely to primary care in the community compared to those cared for by the hospital diabetic clinic (Hayes & Harries, 1984).

If all diabetics were looked after solely by general practitioners, undoubtedly some would be cared for by doctors without a real interest in the subject. If all diabetics were cared for solely by the hospital, then diabetic clinics would be overloaded leading to difficulties maintaining standards, and the expertise and interest in the community would probably decline. Perhaps the way forward lies with a physician with an interest in diabetes based in each district general hospital providing a nucleus of expertise and sharing care with interested general practitioners. This would reduce the strain on hospital clinics, stimulate interest and expertise in diabetes in the community and ensure diabetic patients had a regular review in a specialist clinic. Perhaps general practitioners wishing to provide some diabetic care should have a period of training in the specialty and work for a period in a diabetic clinic to enhance their experience. Their practice nurses would need some specialist diabetic training and they would need a dietetic service.

The practice would need to be able to accurately check the blood glucose, weigh the patient, examine the eyes and record the results. A cooperation card could be used to facilitate communication between diabetic clinic and general practice.

Organisation of Diabetic Care in Hospital

The diabetic clinic is the focal point of diabetic care in the hospital. It needs to be organised to provide a happy, relaxed but efficient environment for seeing patients. The prime objective for a clinic is that the patient returns to be seen again and everything is secondary to that objective. Although achieving good control and all the other objectives are very important, none of these is likely to be achieved if the patient persistently fails to attend. Undoubtedly, the skill of medical care in all specialties is balancing what the patient will accept with what the patient should accept. For example, if the patient says 'I cannot possibly measure my own blood glucose because I am at work all day', the patient might be lost if the doctor were to insist. However, if the patient were introduced to other patients who were monitoring their own blood glucose levels, the situation might be quickly resolved. Attendance at clinic is probably encouraged by avoiding long delays and making the visit worthwhile.

The biggest problem with the diabetic clinic is that time tends to be very limited and perhaps it is best regarded as a place for assessment and the identification of problems, with a little time for education. The major part of teaching, motivating and assessing what has been learned should take place outside the diabetic clinic. A solution we have adopted at my hospital has been a Diabetic Unit. This consists essentially of a group of nurses specially trained in diabetic care, and exclusively devoted to that specialty providing a seven days a week, 24 hour per day service. They staff a unit which can take six inpatients and functions as a day unit. Out-patients visit with or without an appointment and can telephone if they have problems. The Unit is educational first and foremost, so that patients are admitted to the beds only if they are fully ambulant and not requiring parenteral therapy. Those admitted to the acute wards with severely uncontrolled diaebtes are transferred when they are sufficiently recovered and undergo assessment of their self-management. Patients poorly controlled in clinic are referred to the Unit as outpatients and only if this fails to resolve their problems is a short admission considered. Inpatient status does permit more intensive teaching and assessment of where management is failing.

A dietitian is responsible for the Unit and visits twice a day. Patients can be seen at times of their choosing by nursing staff, which may be early morning before school or work, late evening or at weekends. If any difficulties arise for the nurses, medical staff are readily available.

The Unit provides an excellent forum for training nurses and doctors about the practical problems of diabetes, whether they are hospital or community based. It has the great asset of open access and staff/patient relationships are excellent. Patients meet there and discuss mutual problems informally. It is complementary to the diabetic clinic and is quite at home dealing with children or pregnant diabetics. Young children are not admitted to the Unit, but there is close liaison with the Paediatric Department. It is a system that would lend itself to any sizeable district general hospital.

The Future

The future should see more contact between interested primary-care physicians and hospital-based diabetologists, with training programmes in most districts for doctors and nurses covering all aspects of care. The newly qualified doctors of the 1980s know too little about diabetes when at least 1 per cent of the population suffer from this disorder with the prevalence rising. Better organisation of care should also be associated with some time in the medical student curriculum being devoted to the practical aspects of diabetes. We look to improved insulin delivery systems, perhaps suppression of the immunological insult to the islet and methods of enhancing insulin receptor activity. Even with these advances I am sure that diabetic care will focus on helping patients to care for themselves effectively.

References

Andreani, D., Menzinger, G., Di Mario, V. et al (1977). Clinical use of monocomponent insulin preparations. *Proceedings of XIVth International Congress of Therapeutics, Montpelier, France 1977:* L'Expansion Scientifique Française, pp. 9–25.

Baker, J.R., Metcalf, P.A., Holdaway, I.M. et al (1985). Serum fructosamine concentration as measure of blood glucose control in type 1 (insulin-dependent) diabetes. *Br. Med. J.* **290**, 352–5.

Bending, J.J., Pickup, J.C., Collins, A.C.G. et al (1984). Rarity of the dawn phenomenon in diabetics treated by continuous subcutaneous insulin infusion. *Diabet. Med.* **1**, 143A.

Bergman, U., Boman, G. and Wiholm, B. (1978). Epidemiology of adverse drug reactions to phenformin and metformin. *Br. Med. J.* **2**, 464–466.

Blackburn, N.A., Redfern, J.S., Harjis, H. et al (1984). The mechanism of action of guar gum in improving glucose tolerance in man. *Clin. Sci.* **66**, 329–336.

Bolli, G.B. and Gerich, J.E. (1984). The 'Dawn phenomenon'—a common occurrence in both non-insulin-dependent and insulin-dependent diabetes mellitus. *N. Engl. J. Med.* **310**, 746–749.

British Diabetic Association (1982). Dietary recommendations for diabetics for the 1980s: a policy statement by the British Diabetic Association. *Hum. Nutr. Appl. Nutr.* **36A**, 378–394.

Clark, A.J.L., Adeniyi-Jones, R.O., Knight, G. et al (1982). Biosynthetic human insulin in the treatment of diabetes. A double blind crossover trial in established diabetic patients. *Lancet* **ii**, 354–357.

Clark, R.S., English, M., McNeill, G.P. et al (1985). Effect of intravenous infusion of insulin in diabetics with acute myocardial infarction. *Br. Med. J.* **291**, 303–305.

Czyzk, A., Królewski, A.S., Szablowska, S. et al (1980). Clinical course of myocardial infarction among diabetic patients. *Diabet. Care* **3**, 526–529.

Editorial (1984). Dawn phenomena in diabetes. *Lancet* **i**, 1333–1334.

Factor, S.M., Okun, E.M. and Minase, T. (1980). Capillary micronaeurysms in the human heart. *N. Engl. J. Med.* **302**, 384–388.

Ferguson, S.D. and Prosser, R. (1980). Are reflectance meters necessary for home blood glucose monitoring? *Br. Med. J.* **281**, 912.

Francis, A.J., Home, P.D., Hanning, I. et al (1983). Intermediate acting insulin given at bedtime: effect on glucose concentration before and after breakfast. *Br. Med. J.* **286**, 1173–1176.

Geffner, M.E., Frank, H.J., Kaplan, S.A. et al (1983). Early morning hyperglycaemia in diabetic individuals treated with continuous subcutaneous insulin infusion. *Diabet. Care* **6**, 135–139.

Gwilt, D.J., Petri, M., Lamb, P. et al (1984). Effect of intravenous insulin infusion on mortality among diabetic patients after myocardial infarction. *Br. Heart J.* **51**, 626–630.

Hamby, R.I., Zoneraich, S. and Sherman, L. (1974). Diabetic cardiomyopathy. *JAMA* **229**, 1749–1754.

Hayes, T.M. and Harries, J. (1984). Randomised controlled trial of routine hospital clinic care versus routine general practice care for Type II diabetics. *Br. Med. J.* **289**, 728–30.

Home, P.D. and Alberti, K.G.M.M. (1982). Human insulin. *Clin. Endocrinol. Metab.* **11**, No. 2, 453–483.

Hjermann, I., Velve Byre, K., Holme, I. et al (1981). Effect of diet and smoking intervention on the incidence of coronary heart disease. Report from the Oslo Study Group of a randomised trial in healthy men. *Lancet* **ii**, 1303–1310.

Husband, D.J., Alberti, K.G.M.M. and Julian, D.G. (1983). 'Stress' hyperglycaemia during acute myocardial infarction? An indicator of pre-existing diabetes? *Lancet* **ii**, 179–181.

Hypertension Detection and Follow-Up Program (1979). Five Year Findings of the Hypertension Detection and Follow-Up Program. 1. Reduction in mortality of persons with high blood pressure including mild hypertension. *JAMA* **242**, 2562–2571.

Karlsson,K. and Kjellmer, I. (1972). The outcome of diabetic pregnancies in relation to the mother's blood sugar level. *Am. J. Obstet. Gynecol.* **112**, 213–220.

Kennedy, A.L., Lappin, T.R.J., Lavery, T.D. et al (1978). Relation of high-density lipoprotein cholesterol concentration to type of diabetes and its control. *Br. Med. J.* **2**, 1191–1194.

Kesson, C.M. and Slater, S.D. (1979). Smoking in diabetics. *Lancet* **i**, 504–505.

Keys, A. (ed.) (1970). Coronary heart disease in seven countries. *Circulation* **41**, No. 4, Suppl. 1, 1–98.

Kjekshus, J.K. and Mjøs, O.D. (1972). Effect of free fatty acids on myocardial function and metabolism in the ischaemic dog heart. *J. Clin. Invest.* **51**, 1767–1776.

Lauritzen, T., Frost-Larsen, K., Larsen, H. et al (1983). Effect of 1 year of near-normal blood glucose levels on retinopathy in insulin-dependent diabetics. *Lancet* **i**, 200–204.

Lamb, P. (1984). Treating diabetes on a coronary care unit. *Practical Diabetes* **1**, 40–42.

Lean, M.E.J., Ng L.L. and Tennison, B.R. (1985). Interval between insulin injection and eating in relation to blood glucose control in adult diabetics. *Br. Med. J.* **290**, 105–108.

Levy-Marchal, C., Albisser, M. and Zinman, B. (1983). Overnight metabolic control with pulsed intermittent versus continuous subcutaneous insulin infusion. *Diabet. Care* **6**, 356–360.

Liedtke, A.J., Nellis, S. and Neely,J.R. (1978). Effects of excess free fatty acids on mechanical and metabolic function in normal and ischaemic myocardium in swine. *Circ. Res.* **43**, 652–661.

The Lipid Research Clinics Coronary Primary Prevention Trial (1984). The Lipid Research Clinics Coronary Primary Prevention Trial Results. II. The relationship of reduction in incidence of coronary heart disease to cholesterol lowering. *JAMA* **251**, 365–374.

Lockwood, D.H., Gerich, J.E. and Goldfine, I. (eds.) (1984). Symposium on effects of oral hypoglycaemic agents on receptor and post-receptor actions of insulin. *Diabet. Care* **7**, Suppl. 1, 1–129.

Lord, J.M., White, S.I., Bailey, C.J. et al (1983). Effect of metformin on insulin receptor binding and glycaemic control in Type II diabetes. *Br. Med. J.* **286**, 830–831.

Luft, D., Schmülling, R.M. and Eggstein, M. (1978). Lactic acidosis in biguanide-treated diabetics. *Diabetologia* **14**, 75–87.

McGill Jr. H.C., Arias-Stella, J., Carbonell,L.M., Correa, P. et al (1968). General Findings of the International Atherosclerosis Project. *Lab. Invest.* **18**, 498–502.

Maxwell, M.M., Waks, A.V., Schroth, P.C. et al (1982). Error in blood pressure measurement due to incorrect cuff size in obese patients. *Lancet* **ii**, 33–36.

Mecklenburg, R.S., Benson, J.W., Becker, N.M. et al (1982). Clinical use of the insulin infusion pump in 100 patients with Type 1 diabetes. *N. Engl. J. Med.* **307**, 513–518.

Mecklenburg, R.S., Benson ,E.A., Benson Jr. J.W. et al (1985). Long-term metabolic control with insulin pump therapy. Report of experience with 127 patients. *N. Engl. J. Med.* **313**, 465–468.

Nattrass, M. and Alberti, K.G.M.M. (1978). Biguanides. *Diabetologia* **14**, 71–74.

Oliver, M.F., Kurien, V.A. and Greenwood, T.W. (1968). Relation between serum free fatty acids and arrhythmias and death after acute myocardial infarction. *Lancet* **i**, 710–715.

Oswald, G.A., Corcoran, S. and Yudkin, J.S. (1984). Prevalence and risks of hyperglycaemia and undiagnosed diabetes in patients with acute myocardial infarction. *Lancet* **i**, 1264–1267.

Partamian, J.O., and Bradley, R.F. (1965). Acute myocardial infarction in 258 cases of diabetes. Immediate mortality and five-year survival. *N. Engl. J. Med.* **273**, 455–461.

Petersen, C.M., Jones, R.L., Koenig, R.J. et al (1977). Reversible haematologic sequelae of diabetes mellitus. *Ann. Intern. Med.* **86**, 425–429.

Phillips, M., Simpson, R.W., Holman, R.R. et al (1979). A simple and rational twice daily insulin regime: distinction between basal and meal requirements. *Q. J. Med.* **48**, 493–506.

Regan, T.J., Lyons, M.M., Ahmed, S.S. et al (1977). Evidence for cardiomyopathy in familial diabetes mellitus. *J. Clin. Invest.* **60**, 885–899.

Roland, J.M. (1984). Need stable diabetics mix their insulins? *Diabet. Med.* **1**, 51–53.

Santen, R.J., Willis, P.W. and Fajans, S.S. (1972). Atherosclerosis in diabetes mellitus. *Ann. Intern. Med.* **130**, 833–843.

Skyler, J.S., Lasky, I.A., Skyler, D.L. et al (1978). Home blood glucose monitoring in diabetic management. *Diabet. Care* **1**, 150–157.

Sonksen, P.H., Judd, L.S. and Lowy, C. (1978). Home monitoring of blood glucose. Method for improving diabetic control. *Lancet* **i**, 729–732.

Sosenko, J.M., Breslow, J.L., Miettinen, O.S. et al (1980). Hyperglycaemia and plasma lipid levels. A prospective study of young insulin-dependent diabetic patients. *N. Engl. J. Med.* **302**, 650–654.

Tattersall, R. and Gale, E. (1981). Patient self-monitoring of blood glucose and refinements of conventional insulin treatment. *Am. J. Med.* **70**, 177–182.

Taylor, K.G., John, W.G., Matthews, K.A. et al (1982). A prospective study of the effect of 12 months treatment on serum lipids and apolipoproteins A-I and B in Type 2 (non-insulin-dependent) diabetes. *Diabetologia* **23**, 507–510.

University Group Diabetes Program (1970). *Diabetes* **19**, Suppl. 2, 747–830.

Veterans Administration Co-operative Study Group on Antihypertensive Agents (1967). Effects of treatment on morbidity in hypertension: 1. Results in patients with diastolic pressures averaging 115 through 129 mmHg. *JAMA* **202**, 1028–1034.

Veterans Administration Co-operative Study Group on Antihypertensive Agents (1970). Effects of treatment on morbidity in hypertension: 2. Results in patients with diastolic blood pressure averaging 90 through 114 mmHg. *JAMA* **213**, 1143–1152.

Vik-Mo, H. and Mjøs, O.D. (1981). Influence of free fatty acids on myocardial oxygen consumption and ischaemic injury. *Am. J. Cardiol.* **48**, 361–365.

Walford, S., Gale, E.A.M., Allison, S.P. et al (1978). Self-monitoring of blood glucose. Improvement of diabetic control. *Lancet* **i**, 732–735.

WHO Expert Committee on Hypertension (1978). *Report of the WHO Expert Committee on Hypertension*, Tech. Rep. Ser. No. 628, WHO, Geneva.

Index